Skin Deep

SKIN
DEEP

*A Mind/Body Program
for Healthy Skin*

Ted A. Grossbart, Ph.D., and
Carl Sherman, Ph.D.

WILLIAM MORROW AND COMPANY INC.
New York

To Selma Fraiberg:
she brought light to so many
kinds of darkness.

—T. G.

To my mother

—C. S.

Library of Congress Cataloging-in-Publication Data

Grossbart, Ted A.
Skin deep.

Includes index.
1. Skin—Diseases—Psychosomatic aspects. 2. Mental
suggestion.   3. Hypnotism—Therapeutic use.   4. Mind
and body.   I. Sherman, Carl.   II. Title.
RL72.G76 1986   616.5′08   85-21465
ISBN 0-688-04772-6

Printed in the United States of America

First Edition

1 2 3 4 5 6 7 8 9 10

BOOK DESIGN BY ELLEN LO GIUDICE

Preface

Skin Deep is an excellent book that should be beneficial to physicians treating skin disorders as well as to patients having skin problems. It will be especially useful to those unfortunate persons with chronic skin disorders.

The authors realize that the psychological techniques they emphasize, and so carefully outline in their book, are not a panacea but a very useful methodology to be utilized in conjunction with conventional dermatologic therapy. In fact the authors rightly stress that any patient with a dermatitis should first start therapy with a dermatologist. Since the vast majority of dermatoses have an emotional component, whether as a cause, an aggravating factor, or a result, patients will find this book of exceptional value in obtaining an insight into their condition.

The mind and the body function as a unit in both health and disease. Since they cannot be separated into distinct entities, to treat one and not the other is often fraught with failure. A combined therapeutic approach is frequently needed for complete relief from many chronic skin disorders. *Skin Deep* will assist patients in obtaining an understanding of the various techniques and effectiveness of psychotherapy in skin disorders.

It is wrong to consider any somatic disorder merely somatic, or any psychic condition totally psychic. The psychosomatic and the somatopsychic cycles are active in the origins of many skin disorders. Treatment should be directed not only at the skin but at the whole patient—body and mind. He cannot be divided into organic and psychic components for separate therapy. Certain cutaneous diseases should be objectively treated as dynamic, constantly fluctuating adaptations to the stresses and strains to which the patient is exposed both externally and internally.

In treating dermatologic patients worldwide I have encountered emotional tension as the key etiological factor not only in patients with highly technical, stressful occupations in large American and European cities, but in multimillionaire Arab patients I observed in the vast deserts of Saudi Arabia, and also in Dayak headhunters whom I treated in the jungles of Borneo. No one is immune to emotional stress. One's skin is frequently utilized, either consciously or subconsciously, as an outlet for relieving tension.

Psychotherapy is an effective method of treatment in the hands of qualified therapists for dermatologic conditions of functional or organic origin. The introduction of psychological thinking into the treatment of dermatologic and allergic disorders enables therapists to attain results far beyond those obtainable by organic therapy alone. However, major psychiatric problems require the assistance of psychologists or psychiatrists.

It is a pleasure to recommend *Skin Deep* not only to practicing physicians but especially to the innumerable people suffering from chronic skin disorders.

—MICHAEL J. SCOTT, M.D.

Acknowledgments

Most of what I'll be sharing with you comes from a timeless pool of wisdom. These methods for promoting health and growth have been developed independently by different traditions. Each has its own labels and notions of who deserves the credit: from the gods to the human founder of that approach.

My debt to the pool is enormous. I will treat it largely as public domain.

Specific credit is due to some key teachers, supervisors, and advisers who helped me first put a toe in the waters. Drs. Fred Frankel, Robert Misch, Theodore Nadelson, Norman Neiberg, Murray Cohen, and Louis Chase directly, and Sigmund Freud, Ram Dass, Sheldon Kopp, and Milton Erickson secondhand, top the list.

Three key people opened the doors to my work with skin problems. Dr. Fred Frankel, Acting Chief of Psychiatry at Boston's Beth Israel Hospital, provided a thoughtful entree into the world of hypnosis. Dr. Kenneth Arndt, Chief of the Dermatology Department, and Carla Burton, R.N., opened their doors with continuing encouragement. The collaboration of these three provided a fine example of the kind of interdepartmental innovation that has made the hospital an international center for both research and outstanding patient care.

The late Selma Fraiberg helped in so many ways, including

providing a model for turning research into a lively and utterly practical tool for human betterment.

Of course the real experts are the people with the problems. Their creativity and "test flying" of the techniques were the ultimate sources of knowledge. The members of the Boston HELP group deserve special credit.

Richard Liebmann-Smith, author and editor, was not the first to say "You ought to write a book about this." But he followed my "Who me?" reply with incisive advice and guidance. He introduced me to Gloria Stern, who became my literary agent and staunch supporter. Her matchmaking brought Carl and me together, and then brought the two of us to Maria Guarnaschelli, senior editor at William Morrow and Company. Maria made it all happen from there.

Kathryn Nesbit of the Reference Department of the Countway Medical Library of the Harvard Medical School did the computer bibliographies, and Dottie Moon the remainder of the library research. Karen Lemieux prepared the manuscript with amazing precision under pressure.

Colleague Dr. Richard Pomerance was a constant source of support and intriguing suggestions.

Psychology Today's Virginia Adams and Christopher Cory shaped and published the first article. The warm response it produced was a major boost to the project.

Finally, my wife, Dr. Rosely Traube, and sons Zachary and Matthew provided the bedrock of love and encouragement.

I spend much of my professional life convincing people that they can live their dreams. The right people helping and an enormous amount of work is all it takes. My deepest thanks to all those who helped me take my own advice.

Contents

Introduction

I am a clinical psychologist: people knock on my door because they are in emotional pain. So you may well wonder what my name is doing on a book about skin disease.

Emotions cause many skin problems and aggravate others. Hundreds of people have been helped by psychological approaches, often after years of frustration and disappointment with conventional treatment. I have written this book to help you.

Don't get me wrong. Dermatology has made remarkable strides in recent decades, with the advent of high-tech aids like lasers and cryosurgery, and new wonder drugs like steroids and vitamin A derivatives; many skin sufferers have been cured by their physicians.

Yet many have not. And if you have brought your persistent eczema, your stubborn warts, your psoriasis or recurrent herpes to specialists and superspecialists, if all the creams, lotions, and medications have failed to help, you must wonder if there is something else—and ardently hope that there is. This is exactly what I want to share with you.

For the last eight years, I have brought relief to skin sufferers by applying a principle both ancient and often forgotten: the mind and body are one. Sure, the skin is an organ, as physical as your heart or liver, and a rash is as physical as a heart attack. But the skin is also an exquisitely sensitive responder to emotions. Just as stress makes your heart beat faster and your blood pressure rise (and may eventually give you a heart attack), fear can make your skin turn pale, embarrassment can make you blush—and emotional conflicts, anxieties, and other stresses can trigger cr aggravate skin disease. Just as doctors have learned to lower blood pressure psychologically, I can teach you to make the mind your skin's ally rather than its enemy.

If someone had told me early in my career I would someday be a sort of skin specialist, I'd have referred him to a colleague— for psychotherapy. What I'd learned was probably what you've been taught to believe; skin disease meant viruses, bacteria, inflammations, and such medical stuff, and were thus well off the psychologist's turf. I could hold someone's hand while he waited for next year's wonder drug, but that was it.

In retrospect, however, my special calling—and this book— had its first glimmer of life way back in graduate school. The professor in this instance was as formidable in looks as in temper; his seminars featured a student's case presentation, followed by his own ruthlessly critical appraisal of the patient's true problem and the student therapist's dire shortcomings. Here was no sentimentalist.

One evening he presented a case of his own: a consultation with a man hospitalized with severe eczema beyond the help of conventional dermatology. He had put the fellow in a hypnotic trance and had him imagine floating in a pool of soothing oil. Like a leper in the Bible, the man had risen from his bed a day later, his skin clear.

What to make of it? The professor's psychotherapeutic skills were great, but so was his ego. More to the point, neither I nor my fellow students knew anything about hypnosis, and the professor's story seemed to violate everything we'd learned about how psychotherapy works. I couldn't dismiss the case out of hand, but I couldn't fit it into my view of what the mind, the body, and psychology were all about. The truth was there, but I wasn't ready for it.

It was nearly a decade later that I learned about hypnosis, privileged to attend a seminar with an international authority in the field, Dr. Fred Frankel of Harvard Medical School. After six months of training, we started to practice what we'd learned with clinic patients. My first was a woman referred from the dermatology department for severe itching and scratching. Our success was dramatic—and almost immediate.

Beginner's luck or not, I was hooked. I set out to learn as much as I could about skin problems, and to gather experience in working with skin patients. In the years that followed, I developed a blend of psychological techniques, including hypnosis, relaxation, imaging, and the kind of psychotherapy that helps patients understand their conflicts about sex, identity, and relationships. I shared with colleagues my successes in working with eczema, warts, hives, and herpes, and they responded, "You really ought to write this up."

Looking over the medical and psychological journals at the Harvard Medical School library—going back more than a century—I saw that such results *had* been written up. Physicians and psychologists using similar techniques had achieved similar success—*but no one had noticed*. Other professionals had read these case reports and shrugged their shoulders, as I had at the graduate seminar years before. They weren't ready to understand. And the public—the long-suffering patients who *needed* to hear about what had and could be done—didn't even know such scholarly journals existed.

So when I wrote about my work, it was for a popular magazine. "Bringing Peace to Troubled Skin" appeared in *Psychology Today*[1] in 1982—and evoked a flood of letters and phone calls from across America as well as from Canada and Europe. I had obviously touched people deeply. Doctors called in, eager to learn my skills, and share their own, but most of the flood was from people in pain. They wanted—desperately—to learn the techniques I described. They were willing—anxious—to work hard, but they didn't know anyone, psychologist, dermatologist, or Indian chief, who could teach them.

I wrote this book for them and for you.

HOW THIS BOOK CAN HELP YOU

There is nothing magical about this, or any other, self-help book. It will not emit vibrations that heal skin. It is not a textbook, a cookbook, or psychotherapy-in-a-box. It is a workbook—and that means you will have to work. If you use the exercises and techniques herein—the same ones that have helped my patients—you will understand yourself in a deeper way, and learn what conflicts, fears, and needs complicate or cause your skin disease. You will learn how to relieve pain and itching through self-hypnosis and relaxation. You will learn how to turn setbacks into vital sources of energy, and what to do when symptoms simply refuse to let go.

Think of my book as a box full of tools. I've found in my practice that no one uses all these techniques, and most people get maximum benefit from just a few. Which will work for you? I'm a firm believer in each person's ability to find what he or she needs: as you read, feel free to pick, choose, experiment, and discover the tools that work for you.

One piece of advice is basic. No matter what skin symptom you have, *see your doctor first*. Conventional dermatology works for many, and when it does, it works more quickly and more simply than my approach. Skin problems can be symptoms of a general problem; liver disease or diabetes may cause itching, for example. Your doctor will know when to look further.

But above all, remember: this book is only paper and ink; you are the active ingredient, yours the active role. Your skin problem belongs to you. Are you ready to let it go?

PART ONE

The Story
Behind
Your Skin

1

How This Book Can Help

It's easy to think of the skin as a mere wrapping to protect the sensitive organs inside the body. But to understand its problems, you must realize that the skin itself is an organ, just like the heart, lungs, and liver. It is the body's largest organ, in fact—and perhaps its most sensitive.

The outermost layer of skin, the *epidermis*, is constantly renewing itself with cells that move upward from the tough *dermis*, which largely consists of connective tissue. Beneath the dermis, *subcutaneous* tissue stores fat to provide energy and insulation.

Like other organs, the skin plays its part in the complex biological orchestra of life processes. Its sweat glands relieve the body of salt, water, and waste products. With energy from the sun, it converts a cholesterol-like chemical to bone-building vitamin D. Recent research suggests that the skin plays an unsuspected role in activating immune-system cells that protect the body from disease.[1]

What makes the skin unique among organs is its exposed position—up against the outside world. Other body organs can function only in a controlled, protected environment where the temperature never varies far from 98.6°F. It is the skin that maintains this environment, and to do so it must be able to take on temperatures ranging from dry desert heat to bitter cold. It must be exquisitely *sensitive* to its surroundings: when the outside temperature rises, blood flow through the skin must increase and sweat glands must secrete liquid whose evaporation will keep inner temperature from rising too. When temperature dips, vessels must constrict to conserve body heat.

To sense and respond to the outside world, the skin is richly supplied with nerve endings that link it intimately with the body's control center—the brain. Messages from sensors on the skin tell the brain that temperature has dropped or something sharp is in contact with the hand; messages from the brain immediately take steps to conserve heat, or pull the arm back for protection.

Thanks to its close connections with the nervous system, the skin is acutely sensitive to emotional events as well. It turns pale and clammy when we experience fear (the "cold sweat" of anxiety), it blushes when we're embarrassed, and it "glows" when we're happy. Anger, depression, and elation cause subtle but measurable changes in the skin.

MIND AND BODY, SICKNESS AND HEALTH

Actually, *all* body organs respond to emotion, directly or indirectly, and this interconnection of mind and body may be the most important rediscovery (Hippocrates knew it; like many truths, it was often ignored for centuries) of modern medicine. Even conservative physicians now recognize that emotionally stressful events can lay the body open to various diseases, from infection to heart attack. Modern healers prescribe relaxation exercises for high blood pressure and use hypnosis to quell pain that resists the strongest drugs. To prevent heart disease, we're advised to delete not only cholesterol from our diets, but hostility and over-competitiveness from our behavior.

Medical research has linked troubled minds and troubled bodies. In one study, husbands of women who died of breast cancer showed a marked depression of immune defenses during the period of grief that followed their loss.[2] Accumulating evidence links personality type with vulnerability to heart disease and cancer. Another study found that when people visited faith healers, antibody levels rose in their bloodstream.[3] Your emotions, thoughts, and beliefs can make you sick—or well.[4]

Given the skin's intimate bonds with the nervous system, the role of the mind in skin disease should be small surprise. All the more so when you consider that psychologically as well as physically, the skin is your boundary with the world outside, at which every act of love, hate, work, and play takes place. You touch the world and the world touches you through your skin: it is here that you experience pleasure and pain. The skin is at once your most public organ, the face you show all the world, and supremely private territory: baring and caressing of skin is the very image of intimacy.

When something goes wrong with the skin—hives, eczema, warts, or whatever—my experience as a psychologist has taught me to keep the skin's double life, as emotional and physical organ, in mind; to remember that emotional difficulties can cause some skin diseases, and that even when the cause is clearly physical (heredity, infection, chemical irritation), they may trigger attacks or make them more severe.

Let me explain. "Emotional difficulties" doesn't mean "feelings." No matter how painful, feelings themselves cause us less trouble than *our efforts to protect ourselves from them.* When we don't *experience* the pain of difficult events—when we don't feel our feelings—we are much more prone to develop physical symptoms, including skin disorders.

Remember the law of conservation of matter and energy from high school physics? Matter and energy can't be destroyed, but can only change form. Burning can turn wood into light and heat, and pounds of fat can turn into the energy we expend while running. Our minds and bodies are governed by what I call the law of conservation of emotional energy. We can push away the anger we're afraid will get out of control, the sexual urges we've been taught are bad, the emptiness and longing for love that parents withheld. But we can't *destroy* them. The feelings find their own way out to the surface—often through the skin.

Your skin, in fact, leads an emotional life of its own, filled with the feelings you've avoided to protect yourself against pain. Your skin feels *for* you: it cries and rages; it remembers events so painful you've swept them under the rug of consciousness. It punishes you for real or imagined sins. Your skin can't talk in words: its emotional language may consist of warts, or an "angry rash" of eczema, or an outbreak of shingles or psoriasis.

How does emotional turmoil cause, trigger, or heighten symptoms? Researchers are actively exploring this mystery; a key discovery seems to be the body's ability to turn intensely experienced ideas and fantasies into physical realities. (If you *imagine* someone is breaking into your apartment, your body will go into high alert, even panic, just as if the threat were real.)

In a classic experiment, Japanese physicians Y. Ikemi and S. A. Nakagawa hypnotized volunteers and told them a leaf applied to their skin was a toxic plant like poison ivy. The plant was in fact harmless—but the subjects' skin became red and irritated. The same experimenters applied the real toxic plant to other subjects' skin, after telling them it was innocuous. The expected biological reaction did not take place.[5]

A wide range of skin symptoms have been produced—and relieved—experimentally with the focused mental power of concentration and suggestion.[6] As early as 1928, Drs. Robert Heilig and Hans Hoff of the University of Vienna used hypnosis to alleviate outbreaks of oral herpes (cold sores). In an experiment, they could also *trigger* outbreaks in these patients by reminding them, under hypnosis, of the painful events that had triggered them originally (such as a death in the family), and of itching and tingling that usually come just before the sore appears.[7]

Drs. Ziro Kaneko and Noburo Takaishi of the Osaka University Medical School used a similar procedure with hives. Fourteen of the twenty-seven patients they treated made complete or near-complete recoveries; only five reported no benefit. They too could bring the symptoms back with hypnosis, either by suggesting skin irritation directly or by bringing to mind situations that aroused anger.[8]

No, I am not the first to relieve skin problems with psychological therapies. Some two dozen scientific reports, including several large-scale studies, describe successfully treating warts this way.[9] In recent years, more and more researchers have applied these techniques to a wider variety of symptoms. For example, the British physicians Brown and Bettley found that many eczema patients improved markedly when psychotherapy was added to their regular medical care.[10]

WHAT THIS BOOK CAN DO FOR YOU

Rather than dividing illness into "emotional" or "psychosomatic" and "physical," I think of emotions as a *factor* in all skin problems. Emotional difficulties may be the sole cause of few symptoms, but they play a role—major or minor—in the flare-ups of many, perhaps most. Emotional factors sometimes cause, and very frequently can reduce or intensify, itching and pain, even when the physical disease itself remains unchanged. All skin problems have an emotional *impact*, regardless of cause.

How important is the emotional factor in your illness? The more of these questions you answer yes, the more significant the factor:

1. Does your symptom get worse—or better—with emotional turmoil?
2. Is your condition more stubborn, severe, or recurrent than your doctor expects?
3. Are the usual treatments ineffective?
4. Does every treatment work, but not for long?
5. Is your skin worse in the morning, suggesting that you rub or scratch unintentionally at night?
6. Do you have trouble following your doctor's instructions?
7. Do you do things you know will hurt your skin, like squeezing pimples or overexposing yourself to sunlight?
8. Does your distress seem out of proportion to your problem's severity?
9. Do you feel excessively dependent on your dermatologist— or excessively angry with him or her? (Even if the faults are real, are you overreacting?)
10. Does it seem that others notice improvements in your skin before you do? Is it hard for you to acknowledge that your skin is better?

The more of these questions you answered positively, the more likely a candidate you are for my program. But even if most or all of these questions don't apply to you, my psychological approach will offer three important kinds of help:

1. Exercises to help you focus on the hidden role of your emotions in the disease itself. Are they causing, triggering or heightening outbreaks? You'll learn to know yourself and use this knowledge to make your skin better.
2. Techniques to reduce itching, scratching, burning and pain—regardless of their source.
3. A systematic method to reduce the emotional impact of your illness, so you can cope better and suffer less while your skin improves.

Small Changes, Big Effects

A persistent illness reflects a stalemate between the forces of health and disease—that's why symptoms don't get progressively worse, but never get entirely better. Such forces are complex: the cause of your eczema, for example, may be 50 percent hereditary susceptibility, 40 percent environmental irritation, and 10 percent emotional factor. Although the impact of the latter is relatively slight, improvement here can *tip the balance* in favor of health, promoting remission. It's like the way a drooping houseplant comes vibrantly back to life when moved just a few feet into the light or away from the radiator.

If you have recurrent warts, shingles, or genital herpes, for example, you're possibly free from symptoms most of the time: the balance is toward health, with the disease-causing virus held in check by the body's immune system. An emotional upheaval causes a temporary dip in defenses, allowing the virus to come out of hiding and cause an outbreak. You develop psoriasis only if you've inherited susceptibility to the disease; but about two-thirds of the time, what triggers an attack or flare-up is the emotional factor.

You can't change your heredity or eradicate the virus that causes warts or herpes, but the psychological techniques presented here can minimize stress and turmoil and maximize healthy emotions to give you leverage for major improvements. By applying them, my patients have made warts disappear, extended the period between herpes outbreaks (or ended them altogether), banished hives, and made persistent skin infections less severe.

The theory is that we succeeded in focusing the mind, via relaxation and suggestion, to effect tiny changes in blood flow, body temperature, muscle tension, and immune function that made enormous differences in the physical processes that produce skin symptoms.

Symptom Relief

Pain, itching, burning, and tenderness respond particularly well to my approach. Doctors have long noted that these symptoms don't necessarily correspond to the severity of their physical causes. After an injury has healed completely, for example, the pain may persist for years; eczema may remain physically severe, while its itching diminishes. I've taught my patients to use techniques like self-hypnosis and imaging to dramatically reduce pain and itching. Like them, you can learn to harness your imagination to bring cooling, soothing relief from the symptoms that cause you the most distress. You can do this for the most physical of diseases, in the same way that doctors have used hypnosis to quell the pain of cancer and childbirth.[11]

From Body to Mind

That your mind can make your body suffer may take some getting used to, but few people question the reverse connection: the emotional anguish that attends any long-term physical illness. It's a blow to self-esteem to feel so vulnerable, particularly when a disease restricts your ability to live in a normal way and achieve normal satisfactions. You may feel a sense of shame for your weakness: you suffer from feeling your body is not under your control. You may be forced by disease into a childlike dependency; you must look to your doctor for relief, as you once looked to your parents.

Skin diseases have a special power to torment. Appearance-altering illnesses like acne, eczema, psoriasis, and ichthyosis can promote extreme shame and isolation. Vitiligo, for example, is a depigmentation of the skin, purely a cosmetic problem in most cases, causing neither itching nor pain. Yet a study of patients found 40 percent reporting depression at their appearance.[12]

Transmissible diseases heighten a sense of personal badness or dangerousness, as genital herpes illustrates all too dramatically. In a survey of herpes sufferers, 84 percent reported depression, 70 percent a sense of isolation, and 35 percent impotence or diminished sex drive.[13] None of these are physiologically related to the disease; all represent a profound emotional reaction I call psychological herpes.

The root of its special turmoil, suggests psychiatrist Ted Nadelson, is the sense of "dirtiness" (absolutely without basis in fact) that attaches to skin disease, but not to ulcer or heart attack. Dirt, according to Freud, is "matter in the wrong place" (contrast drinking a glass of water with spitting into it and then drinking). Your skin is the boundary between the inside of your body and the outside world; a sore or eruption seems, in fantasy, as if these internal contents have spilled out—they are out of place and thus dirty. Because this kind of "dirt" cannot be washed off, it seems particularly loathsome.

From toilet training onward, we're taught to associate "clean" and "dirty" with good and bad. The saying that cleanliness is next to godliness expresses a deeply rooted belief. The "dirt" that appears in skin disease feels like the dirty, shameful part of ourselves, the impulses that we've been taught to keep contained within. It seems as if we cannot control our bodies or our impulses, or hide the deep parts of ourselves that others manage to keep out of sight.[14]

Skin diseases are no more dirty, shameful, or reprehensible than pneumonia or diabetes, of course. Were we purely rational beings, any disease would seem a bodily problem to be treated and survived, no more and no less. But *none* of us are such beings: our emotions are what make us human, and shame, guilt, anger, and despair are part of the heritage.

The physical toll of skin disease is bad enough, and its emotional turmoil compounds the pain. If you're like many of my patients, you're adding a totally unnecessary layer of misery with self-criticism. "It's minor medically—I must be psycho to make such a big deal out of it," they say. "I don't have such a bad case, but I'm so depressed. My parents always complained I was 'oversensitive'—I guess they were right."

I'll tell you what I tell them: *If even a minor skin disease is making you feel depressed, anxious, or otherwise upset, you're just reacting normally.* Spare yourself the added burden of blame for feeling what anyone else would feel in your place.

Different skin diseases carry their own brands of torment: a person with genital warts may brood about contagion, but he's spared the visible stigma that bedevils the woman with acne. Severe itching is invisible to others, but can become a life-consuming obsession. Here are the seven emotional reactions I see most often:

1. *"I'm bad; no one will love me."* People with skin diseases commonly reproach themselves with terms like "outcast," "leper," "damaged goods," "reject," "disgusting," "pizza face." They feel defective and hopeless; the more visible or contagious the problem the worse the feeling. "No one will want to go out with me—I'll never get married—my chances at normal life are shot," they think.

2. *"I hate the world; I hate myself."* People with communicable diseases like venereal warts and herpes often harbor rage against those who infected them: some become bitter and cynical about the opposite sex, and a few even transmit the disease intentionally. People with psoriasis and ichthyosis, which are hereditary, may rage against their parents. Pain, itching, marred appearance, and disability can provoke a deep anger against the disease and the world of "normal" people. The anger sometimes turns inward. While few people are at risk of killing themselves, a far more common danger is *fractional* suicide. Despairing sufferers kill off little pieces of themselves—a passion is allowed to cool; a hobby is abandoned; an opportunity for pleasure or success is ignored.

3. *"I'm so alone."* Skin sufferers frequently withdraw from social life, casting themselves as lepers who have no place among decent folk, and the insensitive or irrational reactions of others compound the problem. It is particularly common to feel, "No one who doesn't have my disease can understand how I

feel." A Swiss study of people with a range of skin disorders found their circle of friends diminished dramatically; they typically made no new friends after the disease appeared. Many people resigned from clubs and organizations when symptoms started, exchanging social activities for solitary pursuits like walking, stamp collecting, and reading.[15]

4. *"My life is hopeless."* Powerless to change their skin symptoms for the better, many people extend a feeling of despairing impotence to all the challenges of adult life. A lengthening history of unsuccessful treatments deepens this sense of hopelessness.

5. *"It's all because of my skin."* Sufferers often blame their skin disease for everything that's wrong with their lives, bathing "the good old days" in a false glow. A man may believe his social isolation is caused by his eczema, when actually he was withdrawn and fearful of dating long before the symptom became troublesome. Preexisting sexual problems, depression, and anxiety are easily lumped together as the fault of the illness, making it doubly difficult to relieve either skin symptoms or real life problems.

6. *"My disease means . . ."* The search for meaning in misfortunes is human and healthy, but allowed to run wild it causes trouble. Abetted by well-meaning friends and family who suggest, "Everything happens for a reason," many skin patients falsely conclude they're being punished for their sins or victimized by malevolent fate.

7. *"It's an avalanche."* In any disease where emotions play a role, anxiety about recurrences or flare-ups can trigger exactly what is feared: it's a self-fulfilling prophecy. Panic about the illness can infect the whole sense of one's life—it may seem that everything is caving in at once. Less dramatically, the anxiety-disease-anxiety cycle can simply prevent symptoms from getting better.

Only the most philosophical of us can hope to ride through illness without emotional turmoil. The more you learn to understand these feelings, however, the better control you can achieve over them. Even while you're still in pain, tormented by itching, or unavoidably aware of your marred appearance, you can shed some of the self-blame, fear, and anxiety that seemed to come with the territory.

One secret is getting to know your emotional weak points. Anyone may suffer embarrassment when he or she must present a blemished face to the world, but a person whose self-esteem is low to begin with will endure a special distress. If your upbringing made you uncomfortable about your sexual needs, genital warts or herpes may provoke an extra dose of agony. Knowing *why* you suffer your larger-than-life torments is the first step toward cutting them down to size.

Understanding your conflicts, needs, and fears—understanding *your skin's emotional life*—is also the most important first step toward controlling the psychological factors that cause, trigger, or aggravate your disease. For this reason, self-diagnosis is the groundwork of my program. In the chapters to follow, you'll learn why "know yourself" is a key part of a prescription for healthier skin.

2

Listening to Your Skin

Close links with the nervous system make your skin highly sensitive to emotions; it can be more in touch with your innermost needs, wishes, and fears than your conscious mind. *You* may not be aware that tomorrow's conference is causing deep-down anxiety, but your skin is expressing that tension in hives or an outbreak of acne.

A persistent skin symptom is often a message from the inner you—a call for help. Deciphering this message is like learning to interpret another person's "body language" instead of simply listening to his words. What is your skin trying to tell you? It is part of a complex mind-body organism, designed above all for survival. And survival for any organism means satisfying basic needs. Skin symptoms may irritate, inconvenience, even torment you, but they are often attempts to obtain what you need, biologically and emotionally, in order to flourish.

Emotional needs sound intangible next to biological needs (love vs. food and water), but they're scarcely more negotiable, and it's hard to tell where one ends and the other begins. In a famous study, the French psychoanalyst René Spitz observed infants in an orphanage. All their biological needs were apparently met: they were fed, clothed, and kept warm. But they received no love— they were seldom picked up and fondled as more fortunate infants in loving families are. Many of these babies, Spitz observed, did not grow properly. Without the vital nutrient of love, some physically withered; some died.[1] Other studies have confirmed the necessity of love and cuddling for healthy development. Institutionalized babies, for one thing, are far more prone to eczema than others.

Our needs are most dramatically visible in our totally dependent first years, but they persist throughout life. Just as we never outgrow needs for food, water, and warmth, we always need three kinds of emotional nourishment: *love, respect,* and *protection.*

Love is the emotional equivalent of food, the nurturing gift of a world that supports life. We also need *respect;* love, food, and the rest given *as we require them,* not arbitrarily or impersonally. As adults, the respect of family and friends confirms us as independent human beings who deserve recognition. We need *protection* from emotionally intense extremes as well as extremes of temperature, if we are to grow and flourish. In time, just as we learn to keep ourselves comfortably warm or cool, we learn to protect ourselves against emotional overload.

The world being imperfect, there is often conflict between what we need inside and get from outside, and it is at the boundary— the skin—that this conflict is acted out. Unmet needs obey the law of conservation of psychic energy: the longing for nurturing love at six months or adult recognition at forty won't simply disappear if unsatisfied. We try and try again, first one way, then another, to get what we need. The desperate route of last resort is the physical symptom.

If a baby is starved for love, for example, it will cry for more. If this doesn't work, it may have a tantrum, then become lethargic—or finally develop infantile eczema. The emotional pressure and pain of its frustrated need strains the baby's young body till it breaks down at its weak point. With eczema, the whole body cries through the skin.

Even skin problems that strike previously healthy people in their later lives may have psychological roots in the long-ago days when needs were strongest. In fact, indications are that the roots of such ills may extend back before birth: infants born with allergies or eczema may be at risk from heredity, or may have been subjected to unusual prenatal stress.

Troubled skin is like a loyal but not very bright servant who refuses to quit until it accomplishes what it was ordered to do. The process is hardest to stop when it works, even a little. One of my patients, starved of emotional nurturance as a child, had carried into adulthood an insatiable need to be cared for. Her raw, inflamed skin got the soothing attention her organism craved, but at a high price: normal life was impossible.

Until you hear what your skin is trying to tell you, it will just repeat its message—the voice of your deepest needs—over and over. Try to shut it up with medications or stoic indifference, and it may simply cry louder. The alternative is to give your inner self what your skin is asking for. And when that is impossible, to face the pain of frustrated needs squarely, and work to resolve it directly. A tall order, but the first step is one you can take right now.

That is to think about your skin problem in a new way. Peel off the medical label you've been living with—forget you have "shingles" or "hives" or whatever—and consider your illness as a *symptom* of a deeper need. Don't let the physical nature of your symptom, visible, tangible, and painful as it is, obscure the emotional factor that may be more important. Your shingles may have more in common, on this level, with your neighbor's hives than with another case of shingles.

The first step in treating the problem under your skin is re-labelling it in psychological terms. I find it most useful to ask *what your troubled skin is trying to do for you.* Is it trying to satisfy the primary needs of love, respect, and protection, or to resolve problems that arose when these needs were frustrated long ago? To start relieving your skin of its emotional burden, you must identify and understand the *tasks* it is laboring to accomplish.

1. YOUR SKIN IS CRYING OUT FOR LOVE AND PROTECTION

The satisfaction of basic emotional needs is so important that we're designed with biological mechanisms to get the job done! There's something inborn that makes us smile at a baby and want to cuddle it. The vast majority of parents do the best they can in nurturing and protecting their children. But human beings are imperfect, and life in the world is difficult. A mother may be the victim of a poor upbringing that crippled her ability to give love. A major upheaval (death in the family or abandonment, perhaps) may deny the baby adequate love and protection. Many families are so impoverished that the struggle for bread makes proper nurturing impossible.

A failure to satisfy these early needs leaves an emptiness within. A voracious emptiness, in fact; an emotional black hole that absorbs all the love, respect, and protection we get later on, and cries insatiably for more.

We keep on trying to fill this emptiness with misguided attempts at self-feeding or self-mothering. We buy ourselves new clothes when we're down; we buy "the right kind" of car or a shampoo that TV commercials say will bring us love. The alcoholic and drug addict are enmired in a doomed and destructive attempt at self-feeding. They require the chemical illusions of love, protection, and respect because they still suffer from an early deprivation of the real thing.

Joan [2]

When Joan B. was an infant, her father abandoned the family. Her mother, emotionally devastated herself, simply could not provide her baby with sufficient love and nurturance. Lacking the words to express her needs, the infant Joan let her skin do the talking: severe infantile eczema gave voice to her pain and loneliness.

The adult Joan, married and a mother, remained plagued by troubled skin, which continued to cry out for the love and attention absent from her earliest years. It cried stridently enough, at times, to require hospitalization. Being in the hospital, for Joan, meant a return to childhood: she was exempted from the demands and responsibilities of daily life, and "mothered" by nurses who bathed and comforted her tormented skin. Even lesser episodes treated at home enabled Joan to self-mother her skin with cortisone creams and special baths.

A flare-up of eczema, significantly, was particularly likely when a temporary abandonment by her husband—a short business trip, for example—reawakened the devastating loss inflicted by the first man in her life.

Joan worked with me long enough to see brief but quite dramatic improvement. Her therapy came to an abrupt end, however: I went on vacation—for her, a repeat of her father's abandonment—and she fled.

2. YOUR SKIN IS RAGING

Anger is the reaction we often feel when our fundamental emotional needs are not met. When couples fight, I've found that 85 percent of the time the anger behind the discord means: "You don't love me, or protect me, or respect me as a person."

Anger is a normal, healthy reaction, but many of us were taught to deny it. Anger isn't *nice*, so if we express anger, or even feel it, then *we* aren't nice. Parents often have a repertoire of subtle ways of telling their children that they aren't acceptable when angry. Mixed messages from parent to child are particularly confusing—and far from uncommon. At an extreme is the parent who beats his child, giving him much to be angry about while intimidating him into denying his anger. The child may also be so turned off by his parent's fits of rage that he disowns any of his own similar feelings.

Instead of feeling our anger and expressing it as directly as possible (recognizing our rage in an unfair boss without punching him in the nose), we often suppress it or turn it inward. Suicide and fractional suicide—self-destructive behavior like alcoholism, accident proneness, relinquishing pleasures that make us feel alive—reflect anger turned against the self. Anger is a common ingredient of depression.

The "passive aggressive" person means to feel no anger at all, but has developed the sophisticated ability to arouse it in others. He satisfies his need to vent anger by provocative behavior that infuriates; not only does this strike out more effectively than any display of temper, it induces others to feel his anger for him.

Unfelt, unexpressed anger is the most common psychological mechanism beneath troubled skin. Since it is unsafe or unacceptable to feel anger toward others, the skin is elected to take a beating—another way that anger is directed against the self.

Alternatively, the skin becomes the voice of anger that the child within the adult was forbidden to express. A red, *angry* rash tells the world what its owner cannot: "Look how I've been brutalized." It may represent a visual assault or an underground attempt at revenge against an indifferent parent—a way to let the world know the truth beneath the calm facade.

George

Twenty-two-year-old George M. came into my office with an edgy, guarded look, and a right hand covered with layers of painful red warts that had resisted the best efforts of dermatology for months. They had appeared mysteriously, had worsened inexorably, and seemed determined to stay.

George's early life had lacked nothing but warmth. His parents were responsible and dutiful, but they both had to work, leaving the task of caring for him and his four brothers and sisters to Grandma, an efficient but undemonstrative woman.

George recalled no resentment over his chilly upbringing. In fact, he felt no resentment about anything. The last year, he admitted, had been difficult: his neighborhood buddies had departed, one after another, for the army, for jobs in the Sunbelt, for marriage. He had enjoyed his job until he was arbitrarily shifted to another part of the plant, six months ago. Was he angry at the treatment? Not at all. But it was then that the warts had appeared.

Early in therapy, it became clear that George had never quite outgrown the common childhood fear that anger is dangerous: if he was angry at someone, he'd hurt him. The losses of everyday life failed to elicit the anger they deserved. Instead, anger was turned inward, where George himself would suffer but do harm to no one else.

It was significant that as George's warts vanished and he worked through his inability to express anger, he developed a lively interest in the sport of boxing. When his hands could strike out legitimately, his skin no longer had the task of expressing his rage.

3. YOUR SKIN IS TRYING TO CONTROL

A child can receive abundant love, yet still suffer frustration of another essential need: respect. From our earliest days, we must be acknowledged as independent beings, not mere extensions of our parents. Our own selfhood must be respected and the boundary that sets us off from the rest of the world must be recognized.

When parents give love and attention on their own schedule, according to their own needs, they withhold this respect. A classic example is the mother who forces a sweater on her child when *she's* cold and hands the child a glass of milk when *she's* thirsty. The father who arranges every detail with the injunction that "father knows best" is doing the same thing: refusing to respect the autonomy of his child.

Children who are constantly bulldozed by their parents will often fight back. The stubbornly independent child who digs in her heels and automatically says no whenever someone else says yes, who insists on doing things her way on principle, wastes a lot of energy turning daily life into a series of battles. The desperate quality of her stubbornness suggests a life-and-death struggle. She fights to secure the boundaries of herself, to protect the basic integrity of her soul.

People not given respect as children may spend their later lives turning the tables on the world. From the fear of being controlled may come the passion to control others. Some turn into bulldozers like their parents. Others develop a repertoire of ways for getting others to do what they want indirectly, and often are labeled *manipulative*. This pejorative term is unfair because it ignores the underlying struggle to maintain integrity as an autonomous human being. "Manipulative" people are desperate victims as well as victimizers.

In the effort to control the world around them, they may employ argumentative verbal arts and such indirect arm twisting as flirtatiousness, intimidation, or guilt. Chronic or recurrent skin problems can easily be part of this arsenal.

Peter

Peter F., a thirty-seven-year-old laboratory technician, was allergic to nearly everything, a fact none of his friends or family could ignore. The kids wanted a dog? Peter was allergic to dogs. A drive into the country? He was allergic to pollen and field-grass. His wife wanted to go to a French restaurant for their anniversary. Sorry, cooking smells made him break out in a rash.

It was irritating, but no one could get really angry. After all, it wasn't Peter's fault. He was agreeable as could be: "I'd love to, but my allergy" was his inevitable response to other people's plans.

In therapy, I learned that Peter's mother had also had allergies. She was a fragile woman who loved her son but had found it hard to cope with his independence, and kept a tight rein on his behavior. "Control or be controlled" was the lesson Peter's early life had taught him. As his mother had ruled his childhood, Peter tried unconsciously to control the adult world with his allergies. As ever, it was a hollow victory. Peter was more thoroughly controlled by his allergies than anyone else.

In the course of therapy, Peter's skin allergies disappeared entirely. He remains rather controlling verbally, but his sense of humor about it makes him easier to live with.

4. YOUR SKIN IS PLAYING SEXUAL POLICEMAN

For the infant, the satisfaction of primary needs is an immediate, primitive urge—"I want it now!" As we get older, we learn to defer gratification, to ask for things nicely rather than reaching out and grabbing them. The ability to temper and postpone our urges is one thing that distinguishes humans from lower animals.

It is possible to learn the lesson too well, however. The internal policeman that restrains us from grabbing immediate gratification (what Freud called the "superego") can grow so strong that it forbids the satisfaction of perfectly legitimate needs and desires.

Some of us are taught, by parents' examples and reactions, that needs themselves (particularly bodily needs) are bad. The needs won't go away; no matter how repressive our upbringing, something within us strives blindly for love, respect, and protection, with the frequent result a stalemated conflict between inner needs, outer realities, and the "policeman" conscience. In a common version of this stalemate, efforts to get what's wanted and needed are paralyzed by indecision and anxiety.

The conflict may also be played out in the body, where the skin plays policeman to the "criminal" heart. And what the skin often polices are sexual wishes. When the heart says "I want mine now," the skin says "It's bad to want that. You're too greedy, too sexual." Because mature sexuality is all mixed up with our feelings about ourselves, our autonomy and relations with others, it is a prime target for conflict.

The skin is well suited to resolve such conflict. A major skin problem is an effective turn-off, a flag that says "Count me out sexually." Bad skin can also be a protective barrier against the threats and anxieties posed by dating and sexual intimacy.

Derek

A bright, dapper young lawyer, Derek K. had a profound fear of putting his whole heart into anything—the legacy of an emotionally deprived childhood. He maintained a dispassionate, cool posture toward his life; his relationship with his live-in lover was best described as "slightly committed." What brought him to my office was persistent recurrences of genital herpes.

It didn't take much detective work to discover a distinct pattern: the illness flared up whenever he or his lover was out of town. He himself quickly grasped that he'd been unconsciously asking the virus to help him resist the temptation to seek other sexual involvements. Once he became ready to make these sexual decisions on his own, his recurrences ended almost completely.

5. YOUR SKIN IS TRYING TO REWRITE HISTORY

A persistent or new skin problem is often the echo of a battle that was lost decades before, the lasting legacy of childhood with parents who, despite their best intentions, were unable to provide the love, respect, and protection their children required.

When a major chapter in development turns out badly—a cold, distant parent fails to support emotional growth with nurturing love, for example—there's a powerful drive to rewrite history, to replay the same story, this time with a happy ending. It may sound irrational, but it actually reflects the indomitable life force that ceaselessly strives to get what it needs—the same force that drives blades of grass up through the pavement in search of the sun.

Oscar

This was clearly the process that trapped Oscar G., a computer programmer in his late twenties, in an unending series of eruptions of hives. Oscar's mother loved him warmly and well when he was a young child, but when her six-year-old little boy started turning into an independent little man of the world, she simply withdrew. For whatever reason, she could not be as loving to a growing child as she had been to a toddler. It was then that Oscar had his first outbreak.

The adult Oscar fell into a repetitive pattern: he always chose girlfriends who were affectionate and supportive in the early days of their relationship, but cooled off rapidly when he started to act confident and autonomous. Then would come another allergic attack. It was as if Oscar had to reset the stage of his first defeat, so the story could be reenacted—this time, however, with no withdrawal, and no frustrated need for love. Of course, the same unhappy ending was assured by Oscar's choices: young women who resembled his mother—and behaved as she had.

Oscar's skin settled down considerably after some short-term work with me. In longer-term therapy with another therapist, he's continuing to make good progress in his relationship difficulties.

6. YOUR SKIN IS SUFFERING FOR LOVE

Nobody rescues you when you're swimming. If a child learns that the world supplies love, protection, and support only when she's suffering, she may unconsciously conclude that pain is the ticket to getting what she needs. A darker version of the process takes place in the mind of an emotionally or physically abused child: she learns that the ones who love you are the ones who hurt you, and comes to expect an inevitable link between love and pain.

The pairing of love and pain causes no end of trouble in later life: chronic losers, the accident-prone, and those who fear success are among its victims. The early lesson that love can be found amid pain and abuse is the story underlying masochism.

A chronic skin problem surely causes its victims enough suffering to qualify for anyone's support. When love and hurt are paired, the skin can take a very serious beating.

Lorna

Lorna D. was a real puzzle to her dermatologist. The deep sores on her chest, stomach, and legs resembled no disease he'd ever seen. She could recall no contact with any irritant that could have produced the lesions.

Discussion of Lorna's childhood revealed scars of a different sort. Her parents seemed to regard her healthy growth and development as an insult: it brought out the worst of their abusive tendencies. Only when she was confused and unhappy—or physically ill—did they come through with even minimal caring and support.

"Pain brings help" was the lesson Lorna had learned in growing up. During an intensely stressful period—the breakup of her marriage—she called for help the only way she knew how: she had damaged her skin herself, Lorna finally admitted, scarring her body with hair pins.

Lorna is still in psychotherapy, with far to go. With a strong commitment to therapy, however, the odds of success look good.

7. YOUR SKIN IS LOYAL

Our personalities normally evolve like a mosaic: imitating bits and pieces of persons who have affected us, we build up an "internal library" of styles, gestures, and attitudes to be integrated into our own selves. This is a healthy way to form links with those we love and admire. In a tone of voice or a phrase, our mother or father may remain alive throughout our lives.

We often remain loyal to our parents in other ways, adopting their view of us, trying to be what we were in their eyes. This can be a positive process: when our parents thought well of us, loyalty to that view means self-esteem and accomplishment.

But it is as possible to remain loyal to a negative view, to identify with the notion that we are ugly if our parents apparently saw us that way and dressing and acting in a way to make that vision come to life. A disfiguring skin problem can easily be enlisted in this strategy.

Similarly, the normal, healthy process of identification with parental traits can lead to trouble. When a parent is emotionally inaccessible or has vanished, the identification process may take on a desperate, rigid quality: the only way to feel loved is to "become" the parent.

Children are shrewdly perceptive in identifying and identifying *with* what's truly important to their parents. If Dad is a Yankee fan, developing a strong interest in the team will be a good way to get positive attention. Similarly, if he devotes a lot of time and energy to the care of his hives, the message is easily conveyed that hives are the key to closeness.

Some families have picnics together, while in others, treating their damaged skin has assumed the task of keeping everyone close. Certain skin problems do have a hereditary component—psoriasis is one. Pseudoheredity can exaggerate this biological factor, however, turning predisposition into certainty. The "pseudo" in pseudoheredity is evident when the illness is handed down from a figure who, though influential, is not a biological parent. Colleagues Fred Frankel and Robert Misch successfully treated a man with this problem:

Frank

At thirty-seven, Frank was a lonely, isolated man. He was desperately shy, and the severe psoriasis that had bedeviled the most recent fifteen years of his life didn't improve his social skills or feelings about relating to others.

The disorder had developed shortly after Frank left college. He recalled that time as particularly painful because it meant leaving the one man who had ever been supportive and fatherly—his choirmaster. It wasn't until late in his therapy that Frank remembered that this man, too, had had psoriasis. By developing the disease (for which he'd no doubt had a hereditary weakness), Frank maintained a close, comforting link with this compassionate figure. It also spared him the risk and anxiety of socializing with others.[3]

8. YOUR SKIN IS REMEMBERING

Normally, we "remember" what happens to us simply by recording words, images, sounds, and smells in part of the brain where it remains accessible to the conscious mind. But when something is so traumatic or overwhelming that it won't fit into one's world view and sense of self, it is simply too hot for that mechanism to handle. Driven by our need for protection against emotional overload, we try to deny it, to sweep it under the psychic rug.

An extreme example is amnesia. When someone is assaulted by a moment too full of horror and pain—the violent death of a friend, for example—a mental circuit breaker may pop and all memory of the scene may disappear from the conscious mind. But we also selectively forget less traumatic experiences (including repeated experience patterns). This happens throughout life, but it is particularly likely with the events that occurred too early to be remembered verbally.

But the memory (and especially the painful emotions that belong to it) will not go away: it implacably finds its way to the surface. Thus originates much neurotic behavior: rather than facing the emotionally distasteful memory that his mother was a selfish, frightened woman, a man may remember the truth about her *in action*, by finding a series of women who treat him in the same fashion. Here is another attempt to rewrite painful history with a happy ending.

An unexpressed memory may be visible in postures and

movements: the way that a man breathes can encapsulate the fact that he was "smothered" as a young child. A psychosomatic symptom may be a symbolic memorial to an event or pattern of events too difficult emotionally to face directly.

Vic

In his book *Hypnosis in Skin and Allergic Diseases*,[4] dermatologist Michael J. Scott describes a veteran airline pilot who developed mysterious herpes blisters on his forehead each time his flight schedule took him over a particular canyon.

In hypnotherapy (psychotherapy conducted in a hypnotic trance), he recalled that the canyon had special meaning for him. There a friend and fellow pilot had died in a crash. He himself would have made the flight had he not been kept home by illness. The herpes outbreaks disappeared as the pilot gradually allowed himself to experience the buried sadness and guilt he felt over his friend's death.

9. YOUR SKIN IS TELLING FORBIDDEN TRUTHS

Although blushing is usually associated with innocent maidenhood, it's something many of us do from time to time. The stereotypical blush occurs when the stereotypical young lady overhears an off-color remark or joke that she, in her innocence, surely cannot understand. She blushes because she *can* understand it: she knows more than she thinks she's supposed to, and the rush of blood to her face gives her away.

By subtle hints and signs, many parents tell children not to be what they are and not to feel what they feel. The need for love and respect is the enforcer—we cover up or face the threat of emotional starvation. If the order to counterfeit oneself becomes a way of life, we learn to hide the truth from ourselves and the rest of the world: a feeling or thought that doesn't fit our self-image vanishes; we refuse to let ourselves feel angrier or needier or more sexually aroused than we're prepared to admit, just as we learned to hide our true selves from our parents.

But once more, nothing in the realm of emotions simply dries up and blows away on command. The truth we deny frequently rises to the surface to speak itself through the body.

As the body's largest and most visible organ, the skin is a natural nominee for the task of truth-telling—as is evident when we blush. A person trained to a personal party line that "everything's fine" may present his inner turmoil only in his ravaged face. Sometimes, as in the case of Sarah, the skin delivers its forbidden truth in symbolic terms.

Sarah

Thirty-year-old Sarah L. suffered her first outbreak of "neurodermatitis" shortly after the difficult birth of her first son. The child had been "colicky," crying incessantly day and night, and her husband, an accountant, made things no better. His response was to withdraw, pretending the turmoil of his household did not exist.

Sarah could not break through her husband's passivity or elicit the support she needed from him. Yet her commitment to being a good wife and a good mother left her with no exit from the situation. Gradually, the rash on her hands grew so severe that it necessitated cutting off her wedding ring: symbolic fulfillment of the taboo but heartfelt wish to be out of marriage and motherhood. Sarah only understood the emotional logic of her dermatitis years later, when she finally gathered the strength and awareness to end her unsatisfying marriage.

10. YOUR SKIN IS TRYING TO STOP TIME

A patient described how her mother received the news that her first grandchild was on the way: "How could you do this to me? You're making me a grandmother—an old lady!" Does that graceless lament strike a familiar chord? Time is the medium in which we realize our dreams, but it is also in time that we suffer loss. As we grow, we grow older; we die.

The losses of time begin early. Older children lose the close nurturing they received as young children. Adolescence brings independence and frightening responsibility.

The fear of time's passage freezes some lives into paralysis. A major trauma may stop the inner clock as we wait for resources to cope. We feel reluctant to close the book on a part of life when our needs were unmet. We won't total up the emotional ledger for an era with a haunting debit still on the books.

All parents feel twinges of regret as their cute youngsters grow up. If they express their regret persuasively, children may unconsciously oblige them by remaining "forever young." A child taught that he won't make it in the tough world of real grown-ups may be immobilized by fear. He may sabotage promotions because deep inside he feels only good enough for a routine low-level job. Out of exaggerated loyalty to his parents, he may unconsciously refuse to make them old by his own adult accomplishments.

There's often a strange, paradoxical youthfulness about such people: they seem excessively girlish or boyish, perhaps dressing the part. The skin's participation in this rear-guard holding action is most clearly visible in the face of a man or woman who suffers from post-adolescent acne, whose "teenaged" skin shows he or she is still grappling with the conflicts of adolescence.

Stella

Warts under her fingernails drove twenty-two-year-old Stella to distraction—and forced her to quit her job as a dental hygienist. So instead of using the income to rent her first apartment, she remained in her parents' home, working as a clerk in a store across the street.

Nor was this the only rough patch in Stella's life. She seemed to have a run of bad luck in relationships: one man after another began as attentive and caring, but soon turned abusive and humiliating.

"I have to live like I'm still in high school," Stella lamented. Not only was it embarrassing to be still at home, life there meant stepping back into her adolescent role as her mother's servant and constantly mediating bickering between her mother and father.

In therapy, Stella quickly realized that her skin was actually stepping in to satisfy both her own and her parents' wishes—stopping the clock to spare her the trials of mature relationships, and her parents the growing-old pangs of watching their youngest child leave the nest. With this realization and hypnotic treatment, the warts quickly vanished.

11. YOUR SKIN IS TELLING THE WORLD YOU'RE NOT PERFECT

The gleam in a parent's eye is the raw material of the child's self-esteem—a solid, healthy sense of his own worthiness. Some parents, however, simply can't take that kind of pride and thus can't nurture self-esteem: their children grow up depressed and down on themselves, unable to experience their virtues and strengths.

Parents who overpraise a child's accomplishments may seem to encourage self-esteem, but the result is opposite when such accomplishments are demanded to shore up the parents' own frail egos. Insistence that she be the perfect daughter, complete with spotless fingernails and straight-A report card, that he be the flawless athlete-scholar son, deny the reality of the child. He and she may grow up feeling that if they're not perfect, they're nothing—and no one is perfect.

Children unable to develop healthy self-esteem may become adults who counterfeit what their parents failed to foster. These are the tiresome characters who insist on telling you how important their jobs are, how smart their children are, how fine their house and car are. The performance has a hollow ring; it's a caricature of true self-esteem.

These people also have a need to subtly communicate that there is much more to them than the carefully cultivated public image. Their skin may be asked to carry the message.

Lance

At twenty-three, he was a very successful New York model. His nearly perfect face, however, was marred by acne that perversely flared up just before major assignments.

Lance was the youngest of a series of brothers, each of whom had been pressed by their mother to fill the emotional gap left by their depressed, alcoholic father. Each had failed. Lance had valiantly tried to be her champion, had excelled in high school sports and even looked the part, but his acne repeatedly surfaced, the weakest link under his heavy emotional burden. While his mother encouraged his success, she also constantly expressed an unspoken reproach: "How can you be so happy, young, and successful when your poor divorced mother is so miserable?" Lance's acne cried out a disclaimer: "I'm not perfect either . . . I hurt."

I saw Lance only briefly as he passed through Boston en route to assignments in Europe. His postcard, several months later, reported good results with the techniques I taught him.

We're all mixed bags of complicated emotional needs, and the skin problem that can be reduced to a single pattern or task is as fictional as the person whose character consists of a single trait. A real rash endured by a real person may involve several of these patterns. In thinking about your own symptom, it's natural to pick out the one or two tasks that seem most relevant. But don't dismiss any as having nothing at all to teach.

Just as these patterns never involve growing or feeling in isolation, most skin disorders are best understood as relationship problems, rather than the illness of one man or one woman. Infantile eczema, for example, typically signifies trouble between baby and mother; in adulthood, a spouse may come to play the mother's role. Your skin disease means trouble at the border between yourself and others: resolving the underlying tasks will require changes in how you interact with them. First, however, you must learn to see yourself as you really are—under your skin.

3

"Why Me?"
The Skin Has Its
Reasons

"Why me?" Probably everyone who's ever suffered a maddening itch or plague of warts has asked that question. It can be far more than a cry against fate. Beneath it lies "Who am I?"—a riddle that will lead you to a fuller understanding of your skin problem, and ultimately to relief. It was Hippocrates, father of medicine, who said, "It is more important to know who has a disease than what disease he has."

You already know who you are? Not likely. Few of us have a grasp of our identity on all its buried levels. The search for self-knowledge is a lifetime task that goes beyond psychotherapy: it wasn't Freud but an ancient Greek philosopher who commanded, "Know thyself."

Will self-knowledge heal your skin? It's not that simple, but the better you know yourself, the more able you'll be to confront your emotional needs with your head and heart, freeing your skin to carry on its normal physiological duties. And the better you'll cope with the psychological burden of problem skin.

This kind of self-knowledge—discovering what your skin is trying to do for your emotional tasks—is a special challenge. The same fear and pain that kept you from facing them in the first place keep your naked need for love, respect, and protection deeply buried. Don't expect your inner self to yield up its secrets without a struggle.

You've seen a minor-league version of this struggle if you've ever hunted in vain for the vacuum cleaner on a day when you didn't really want to clean. Your heart wasn't entirely in the search: you were the hider and the seeker simultaneously. A similar process may keep a word on the tip of your tongue but tantalizingly out of your conscious grasp. There's something within you that doesn't want the word to be found.

Similarly, when you look within to discover your deepest needs and feelings, you will find the truth in spite of that part of you with a stake in keeping that vulnerable side hidden. I recall one patient who grew up with the "I'm-tough-and-I-don't-need-any-thing-from-anyone" worldview. He had suppressed his need for love until eczema, which required tender care, voiced it for him. Before he could change his life to satisfy these needs directly, he had to accept them. And this meant wrestling down the stalwart (but actually terrified) guardian of a macho self-image.

When you start living with the question "Who am I?" you might expect your pursuit of the answer to be double-crossed by ambivalence—as the inner hider evades your inner seeker. At the outset, commit yourself to pushing toward the deeper truths about yourself, no matter how uncomfortable it gets. Remind yourself relentlessly how much you can gain by finding what you have hidden.

Once you get started, you'll probably find the pursuit of self-knowledge less a trial than an adventure. Many people who begin psychotherapy (a guided, intensive quest to know themselves) worry about opening a Pandora's box of dreadful revelations. In my experience, however, no one ever wants to go back to the status quo once he or she has turned the corner with major discoveries and the changes they bring. It's not a question of finding out some awful truth about yourself, but realizing new dimensions of your personality. This is the essence of growth, the greatest adventure in the world.

Learning to know your inner self and its links with your troubled skin is partly a logical process, like solving a murder mystery, but more a creative exercise, like what an artist does in combining the right colors and shapes to evoke the majesty of a mountain. While logical intelligence proceeds in a straightfor-

49

ward $2+2=4$ manner, creative thinking leaps by association, connecting things that have no apparent link. Thus it is best equipped to grapple with the slippery hidden parts of your personality that you have tried to bury under the logical facade of adult life.

There is no road map to self-knowledge: your path must be your own discovery. The only rule I know that applies nearly universally is this: be alert for surprises. Be ready to learn things about yourself that you always believed untrue—things, perhaps, that contradict a family or personal "party line." Were you always the mild-mannered sister—the one kid who never lost her temper? Do you still think of yourself as a person without an angry bone in her body? Don't turn away if your self-searching finds a deep reservoir of anger. Many people are mild-mannered because they harbor anger that they fear is destructive and dangerous.

Where will you find clues to your inner self? If your eyes are truly open, you'll find them everywhere. Personality is like biology. Just as each cell of your body contains a full set of genes—the inherited code that determines what, biologically, you are—every experience, every introspection, and every interaction with others bears the unique stamp of your personality.

You may find it useful to keep a notebook. I once asked a novelist friend how he invented his characters. For months before he sat down to the actual writing of a novel, he told me, he'd note down random events in the lives of his characters, as they occurred to him. He sketched details of their appearance, imagined quirks of their conversation. Eventually, from these scattered mental brushstrokes would emerge full-fledged (but fictional) human beings. You may discover your inner self the same way. Don't worry about filling pages with grammatical prose. Just jot down whatever you want to hold on to: the same forces that buried your feelings of fear or anger once will work double-time to make you forget them again.

EXERCISES IN SELF-KNOWLEDGE

I can't give you a magic flashlight to find your hidden self, because there isn't any, but I will share some exercises my patients have found exceptionally useful in illuminating those dark corners of the self most often linked to skin problems. To begin with, here is a toolbox of techniques to help you glimpse your inner self through the mask of your everyday life.

What Do You See in Childhood Photographs?

Study these windows on your early world for insight into family politics and key relationships. Who stands with whom? Who's looking at mother—or away from father? Are you staring into the camera or gazing away? What moods are reflected in your family's faces—in your own face? Are you happy? Is there a surprising hint of anger or sadness?

Particularly valuable are family photographs taken just before or after your skin problem started. What's going on here? Remember, we're not engaged in logical analysis. Don't dismiss a mysterious "hunch" about the picture. It may be part of the hidden truth.

One of my patients, whose genital herpes recurred constantly and painfully, used to talk evasively about sexual-identity issues—his doubts about himself as a man. When he brought in a family picture, taken when he was five years old, the issue suddenly became very concrete. There were his three older brothers—brawny kids who looked like junior linebackers. My patient was dressed like a darling little girl, complete with long ringlets. It seemed his herpes recurrences served a necessary psychological function, focusing attention on his penis and providing reassurance it was still there. His parents, apparently, had unashamedly wished it were not.

How Do You Dress?

Your second skin may play out the same scenario as your real skin. Become aware of how you dress. Is the style strikingly older or younger than you really are? Are you more or less formal than your peers? Some people dress to camouflage their sexuality, others to flaunt it. A natty dresser may put high emphasis on his packaging to compensate for doubts about the interior. Others dress so shabbily as to say: "I'm nothing. Don't take me seriously."

The Story Behind Your Skin

Choice of colors is more than simply a matter of style. A woman may dress in "basic black" and other somber shades because her heart is always at a funeral—a clue to depression so obvious that it's easily overlooked. Bright, cheerful colors may reflect an authentically sunny outlook, or an attempt to mask hollow feelings of need. Paradoxically, one can dress in orange for the same reason another dresses in black. Do you *feel* the way you dress?

Some people are constantly "in costume." Let your mind associate freely: are you dressed like a doll, like Cinderella, like Dumbo? Do you look like a bar mitzvah boy, the high school whore, or a '60s leftover?

A patient once described to me her discomfort at being a woman—as she sat in my office dressed in combat boots, baggy pants, and a work shirt. "My camouflage," she said. Discussion brought memories of her fear at her father's interest in her burgeoning sexuality, and her need to hide it from him and from other men. Her long-standing rash (which she abetted by lax skin care) was part of the camouflage, she came to understand.[1]

What Does Your Body Say About You?

In the circles of a tree trunk, you can read not only the age of the tree but its history. Good years and lean years leave their mark in fat rings and pinched, dry rings. Similarly, what we live through leaves its mark on our bodies, on how we stand up to the world and move through it.

Postures, stances, and movement styles express our relationship with others. You've seen people who walk down any street or enter a room as if going through a sniper zone, hugging some imaginary wall, trying to be as close to invisible as possible. The caricature of the dry intellectual, body eclipsed by head, has some counterpart in reality. The development of arms, legs, and upper and lower body reflect heredity, but also the physical and emotional habits of years. Your whole body, not just your skin, tells your story.

Stand in front of a mirror unclothed and look at yourself sensitively. Ignore your skin but focus on your proportions, your shape, your posture. Do you breathe fully or tentatively? Do you look frail, brittle, mechanical, angular? Are you well grounded, solid on your feet, or a bit wobbly? Do you stand as if the weight of the world were on your shoulders?

It's often far easier to see the inner man or woman within the body of another person. Practice these observational skills on strangers in the street; look inquisitively at friends and family. Do you see echoes of their personalities in bodily shape, stance and motion? Do they remind you of anything in yourself?[2]

What Tones of Voice Do You Use?

Become aware of how you sound in conversation. Do you always speak with the same voice? Most of us lapse into different intonations and vocabularies to fit the occasion. This can reveal our identifications—the aspects of other people we've swallowed whole. When we listen objectively and sensitively, we often hear more personality clues in the "tune" than in the words themselves.

Susan D., for example, was a ship captain's daughter, a successful executive who had trouble forming relationships with men. I noticed in therapy that she'd occasionally shift into a brusque, authoritarian voice that said "Don't mess with me"—a captain's voice. This worked wonders in the boardroom, but apparently it frightened her male friends. She'd shift into her father's voice, she ultimately realized, in anxious, intimate situations: a clue that her identification with her father left little room for other men.

On appropriate occasions, your voice may awaken echoes of early life, suggesting tasks you haven't yet resolved. Another patient, Laura B., realized that when she asked her husband for favors, she automatically lapsed into a meek little-girl voice. This realization in turn aroused chilhood memories of standing outside her busy father's study, wondering if she dared disturb him. From this came a clue to the insecurity behind a tense, miserable marriage, and hives that wouldn't go away.

Psychologists have long recognized special times when the unconscious self speaks with particular clarity. If you open your mind to its language, you can learn much.

What Do You Dream About?

Have you left the understanding of your dreams solely to soothsayers and psychoanalysts? While experts are particularly able to grasp their depths and subtleties, dreams can reveal the emotional life beneath the surface to anyone willing to tune in to them. Become aware of your dreams, and take them seriously.

You are the sole scriptwriter, producer, and director of your dreams, so you can begin by accepting responsibility for them. Why do you have your dreams? Freud suggested that dreams reflect wishes—usually in disguised form. If something horrible, frightening, or shameful happens in your dream, don't dismiss it out of hand but ask yourself (it takes courage): "In what sense does this dream belong to me?" This can spark fertile insights into the paradoxical, unacknowledged wishes and fears behind your skin problem.

George M., the young man in the last chapter who was plagued by warts and an inability to express anger, made good strides in releasing his buried emotions, to the point where he rallied himself to begin training for a career he really wanted: driving long-haul trucks. Then one night, he dreamed he was driving a big truck and had an accident in which several people were killed. This clarified to him the danger of his anger, as he'd always imagined it, and helped him understand how he'd immobilized himself to protect others from it.

Everyone dreams; if you think you never do, it's because you don't remember, possibly because you resist the self-knowledge in your dreams. Dreams are freshest and clearest right after you have them, so keep a notebook and pen at bedside to jot them down immediately on awakening.[3]

What Are Your Daydreams and Fleeting Fantasies?

More accessible than dreams, these often express the same unacknowledged wishes. Daydreams may attempt to solve the same tasks you've given to your skin, free from real-life logical constraints. Frequently recurring fantasies and images have special importance.

Often the wish behind the daydream is clear enough: we fantasize about wealth, success with the opposite sex, fame, and achievement. Not as obviously, frequent daydreams on such subjects suggest a feeling that you lack something in those particular departments. People who feel secure in their financial lives may not object to winning the lottery, but they rarely daydream about it.

Unpleasant fantasies of being chased, attacked, or humiliated are paradoxical. What kind of wishes are these? They may represent an attempt to master a particular fear—the same way you go over a near accident for days afterward in an attempt to come to terms with the experience.

You must take the idea of "wishing"—in both dreams and daydreams—broadly. A young man who often fantasized about being chased and shot at, escaping just in time, expressed a wish to *escape*, not to be threatened. It was an attempt to rewrite history: a childhood in which his father constantly took verbal potshots at him and otherwise belittled him. His fantasies also satisfied the wish to be loyal—to a family party line that had cast him as a target. Tuning into the trauma that he repeated endlessly, he took a step toward challenging it.

What Causes Your Flashes of Thought and Flashes of Feeling?

Have you ever walked down the street and felt an unaccountable twinge of sadness or surge of joy? Like daydreams, isolated thoughts and feelings seem to arise out of nowhere, but in fact come straight from your inner self: respect the fact that they have roots and you may come to understand them.

One summer day when I was hiking, I stepped around a rock and was struck by a mysterious wave of sadness. Following the experience back, I realized that in stepping awkwardly I had planted my toes outward, and that had been an eerily familiar sensation. As a child, I recalled, I'd been pigeon-toed, and teased by other kids. I was told to fight the habit by walking with my feet planted outward—the same way I had walked moments before. This helped tune me in to a reservoir of negative feelings about my body—it wasn't what others wanted it to be.

"Hunches" and intuitions that pop into your head are similar. They come out of context with no apparent logic, because they're the product of intuition. No matter how bizarre they are, think of them as metaphorical hints and they may give you insights that logic will take forever to reach.

What Causes Your Slips of the Tongue?

There is much to the idea that "Freudian slips," misplaced or mispronounced words, are messages from the unconscious.[4] Tune in to them, and allow yourself time to wonder what they mean. One of my patients was talking about family pictures when he referred to a "phonograph" of his mother; he came to realize that he avoided looking at her and thought of her as an endlessly nagging broken record.

Similarly, try to be sensitive to the images and recurring phrases of your personal language. A patient of mine constantly referred to each business project as his "baby." When we discussed this, what emerged was striking envy of his pregnant wife, because he himself couldn't bear a child. Another patient expressed himself dramatically: "Here's a real killer for you," he would introduce his stories. "I blasted out of the office . . . but the traffic on the expressway was crushing." He was unaware of the constant undertone of mayhem in his conversation. Bringing this up helped him to appreciate his buried concerns about anger and safety.

What Do You Forget, and Why?

It's a psychological axiom that you forget what you want to. Perhaps one part of you resists actions that are out of tune with your inner needs.[5] Your party line—the idea of yourself you received years ago from your family and still confirm with friends—may blandly assume you like to bowl, that "I'm a person who loves bowling." If so, why is it you never can find your bowling shoes? It may be that your inner self really doesn't care for bowling— and is rebelling against the force of loyalty that allows you to be trapped into doing what you don't much want to do.

Do you often forget your keys, meaning you must bum a ride? Do you leave your wallet home, forcing you to borrow lunch money? It may be that the payoff—perhaps getting others to take care of you—more than makes up for the inconvenience.

What Troubles Do You Have with Other People?

In the reactions of others, we see ourselves. Are you mystified by the way friends and acquaintances react to you? Do they seem unaccountably angry at times? Do they turn morose, or lapse into teasing sexual innuendos? Do they never seem to hear what you're saying? Your buried emotional life may come through your behavior to arouse reactions more appropriate than you know. For example, others may tune in to your hidden anger and respond with anger of their own.

Conversely, you can learn much about yourself by becoming more aware of your own reactions. Does weakness make you especially angry? Duplicity? Arrogance? We often accuse others of things we fear finding in ourselves, and any disproportionate response suggests emotionally charged issues. One of my patients often spent therapy time railing angrily about "freeloaders" and "welfare cheats." It eventually came out that his family had been on relief when he was a child. His indignation was a reaction that walled up the anger, pain, and humiliation of poverty.

Paradoxically, the things that bother you most about friends and family may alert you to what you find attractive. The woman who is first attracted to her husband because of his even-tempered consideration may later complain that he lacks spontaneity and seems "wishy-washy." She may marry a man who is "dynamic and effective," and divorce him because he's "driven" and "insensitive"—*the vices are virtues relabeled.*

Other people can actively assist your quest for self-understanding. Feel free to ask selected friends and family for help. They won't have the same stake in keeping the roots of your problem hidden. Test your perception of yourself against theirs. If someone says something about you that seems farfetched, completely at odds with what *everyone knows* is the "real you," give it a fair, open-minded hearing. Perhaps there *is* something "constantly cheerful," "morbid," or "flirtatious" about you—something with an important bearing on your skin problem.

In a herpes treatment group that I directed, one man announced that he was ready for a serious romantic relationship. Members of the group pointed out that whenever his involvement started becoming more than pure sex or pure friendship, he'd get a herpes recurrence. This was a pattern he couldn't see, but after repeated emphasis by group members—people he'd grown to like and respect—he finally opened himself to this insight about his fear of intimacy and its role in his disease.

PERSEVERANCE

There's more than one road up the mountain to insight, and knowledge of your inner self will emerge in its own time and its own way. Perseverance is a must—not the kind that beats its head against a brick wall, but the kind that is willing to leave things alone for now and come back later. Many people find that they are *ready* for self-knowledge, and as soon as they open their minds to it, they receive insight in an exciting flood.

Try to exploit the times when you're most likely to gain glimpses into your heart. I always found a visit to my Great-Aunt Annie put me back in touch with my childhood. As the last survivor of my grandmother's generation, she made me remember the little boy I once was, and the feelings that made me the man I am now. Her stuffed cabbage was an elixir of memory that awakened the "child" within me!

Many people find physically demanding activities—dancing, running, climbing mountains—loosen their minds and put them into a receptive state where they see the world and themselves with visionary eyes. For me, the days when I can get out of the city and hike in the hills seem filled not only with the magic of trees and rock outcroppings, but a specially lucid state of mind in which knots untie of their own accord, and things I'd found perplexing suddenly become clear.

The key is de-automatization.[6] So much of our lives runs on automatic pilot: anything that takes you out of the rut of custom and habit can help you to see a new world with new eyes.

Stir up your feelings by putting aside the usual security blankets that soften your perception of life. For a few evenings do without alcohol, without the radio, without your cigarettes. Make it a point to try things that take you out of your usual routine—

if you customarily drive to work, for example, take the bus. You may find yourself with eyes open in new emotional territory as well: this is why vacations are so invigorating.

My mother has her own way of dealing with a crisis: any time she has to make a perplexing decision, she shakes up her usual routine by doing things differently. "If my inclination is to zig, I zag," she said. "If I invariably say no, this time I say yes." What you need most in this pursuit of yourself are flexibility and a readiness—an *eagerness*—for surprises.

The journey to self-knowledge is long and full of stops and starts—a frustrating journey if you're anxious for relief of tormenting skin disease. Most of my patients keep up an encouraging pace of progress by combining the exercises in this and the next few chapters with relaxation and imaging techniques (you'll find these later in the book) that aim to relieve symptoms directly.

Working with self-discovery and symptom-relief exercises simultaneously or alternately, my patients find their own rhythm. Going back and forth from one to the other is like walking: one foot's advance enables the other foot to take the next step. Reducing symptoms directly with relaxation, for example, often increases self-esteem (you've shown yourself that you *can* control your body), which gives you courage to face buried needs more squarely. A little improvement begins a cycle of change.

Even when your skin seems firmly on the road to recovery, keep on pushing for more self-discovery. If you simply clip a weed, it may or may not return. You're far more likely to be rid of it for good if you pull it up by the roots.

4

The Animal Test

Self-discovery is an ambitious undertaking, but it isn't all hard work. In fact, the most useful thing you can bring to the task is the spirit of play. When you use your imagination—to day-dream, to tell stories—you step out of the logic-bound world and into a reality of your mind's creation, where you're most likely to glimpse your inner self.

One of the best ways to discover the inner you is actually a game, the sort kids play when they ask each other, "If you had to be an animal, what would you want to be?" The answer to this lighthearted question can be most revealing: it's not always easy to guess who would want to be a tiger and who a cuddly puppy.

A few years back, a psychologist named Cole was leafing through a newspaper magazine supplement while enjoying his Sunday-morning coffee. This issue featured one of those popular quizzes that invite readers to do a bit of instant self-analysis. "What animal would you like to be?" it asked, providing a system to translate answers into a quick personality readout. Such simpli-fied self-tests offer little beyond a few minutes' diversion, but Dr. Cole was intrigued. He worked the notion up into a concise but searching psychological test, which has become known as the Cole Animal Test.

The Cole Animal Test consists of just three questions: What

three animals would you *most* like to be? What three animals would you *least* like to be? Why? It's hard to believe that such a simple exercise can reveal much of the mind's complexities, but I've found that it gives enough information in a few minutes' time to hold its own amid a battery of fancy diagnostic testing. It's a real shortcut to emotional issues.

Since the dawn of human consciousness, we've seen ourselves and our lives reflected in the animals with which we share the earth. Primitive people identified their tribes, their gods, the good and evil forces of life, with totem animals like the bear and the fox. Animals and people who change into animals figure prominently in folk tales and fairy tales. Our deep kinship with animals is expressed in poetry, in the signs of the zodiac, and in our affection for and identification with cartoon characters like Bugs Bunny and Donald Duck.

Animals seem to embody our emotions, fears, and fantasies. The deer doesn't strike us as a shy animal, but as shyness come to life. The tiger of William Blake's famous poem ("Tyger, Tyger, burning bright in the forest of the night") is a symbol of pure energy and rage.

The word "symbol" may have a dry academic sound, but in fact we think in symbols all the time: the ability to do so comes as naturally as the ability to think in words. Symbols express ideas and feelings that otherwise elude us. A man who struggles with pent-up anger that he's afraid to express (or even admit to himself) may find it impossible to say: "I wish I was powerful. I wish I could be angry and unafraid of the consequences." But he can say it all in symbolic form: "I wish I was a tiger." This is the beauty of the Animal Test.

Looking sensitively at fantasy symbols opens up a channel of communication with that inner you that seems determined to remain hidden (that's why I stress becoming aware of dreams and daydreams). The Animal Test is an invitation to daydream in an organized way, to wander like a child in an imaginary world where people change into animals and back again. It's a simple exercise. Just answer these three questions:

- What three animals would you most like to be?
- What three animals would you least like to be?

• Why have you made each choice?

This is not an exercise to ponder and mull over. The three "most" animals and three "least" should come quickly to mind—after all, it's only a game. Just think about it and write them down. Then come up with some simple, direct explanations for your choices.

The work comes when you sit down to figure out the meaning of your answers. Here is more raw material for self-analysis: just as you've been working on the messages carried by your dreams, daydreams, and fleeting feelings, you can look to your Animal Test answers for clues to your inner self.

This test has no simple scoring key, no turn-to-page-163 answers. What kind of person would like to be a beagle, or an eagle? Be alert for surprises.

One of my patients, a doctor's wife, chose only one animal that she'd most like to be—a tiger. A tiger was powerful, proud, and independent, she said. It had claws to strike out. Her answer emphasized concern with two of the primary needs we've discussed: respect and protection. A tiger is beautiful but not cuddly—its beauty is appreciated from a distance. This need for "hands-off" respect may have been the legacy of childhood with an overbearing mother who constantly inflicted her own needs and beliefs with no respect for my patient's boundaries.

The animals she least wanted to be were "worms" and "bugs," because they are "small, helpless, and disgusting . . . they can be too easily stepped on and snuffed out." What was striking here—what is often striking—was how the two sets of answers complemented each other. If the tiger symbolized protection, respect, and effective anger, the worms and bugs suggested a frightening life devoid of both. In my patient's words, these creatures are beneath contempt and unprotected against extermination.

Put very simply, the positive choices in the Animal Test—the animals you'd most like to be—symbolize wishes; the negative "least like to be" choices symbolize fears. For this patient, the wish was for protection and respect: the fear of being contemptible and vulnerable. Positive and negative choices, like wishes and fears, are two sides of the same theme.

A twelve-year-old girl who suffered from warts most wanted to be a monkey, "because they're cute and fun." She least wanted to be a pig ("they're dirty and yucky") or a frog—whose warts are "repulsive." Here, the theme is lovability. The "cute" monkey is lovable and the pig and frog are repulsive—they repel love. The warty frog is a particularly poignant choice, all too clearly reflecting the girl's self-image. I found these choices revealing in a twelve-year-old, on the edge of adolescence. The monkey is lovable in a childlike way, while the pig is repulsive in a down-to-earth, "dirty" way suggesting a frightened view of the sexuality awaiting her. Passing from "cute" childhood to sexual adulthood threatened the loss of love.

Responses rarely pick out a single theme: love, protection, and respect are usually mixed in combinations as unique as the people who take the test. A California woman, a very successful business executive troubled by recurrent eczema attacks, said the animals she'd most want to be were a panther, "strong, smart and fast"; a lion or a racehorse, for the same reasons; or an eagle, which "flies free, has flights of fancy." She least wanted to be a monkey, "because I don't like to be laughed at, or to mimic others," or a giraffe, because it was "awkward and tall. It stands out and looks funny."

The issue of respect stands out in her responses. If you're not thoroughly admirable, you'll be an object of ridicule. Protection is an important subtheme: the lion, panther, and eagle are powerful creatures, well protected with claws and talons. But the choices suggested some conflict in her quest for respect and protection. The giraffe is a large animal and definitely one that stands out—as did my patient in her own field. Yet it was a negative choice: standing out too much—or in the wrong way—makes you laughable.

A subtheme implied here—one that arises frequently—is anger and aggressiveness. The physician's wife similarly chose her "tiger" for its independence and protection, she said, but her emphasis on "claws" brought out its potential to strike out. It was her inability to find the tiger within that brought this woman to see me. Instead of striking back at her infuriating mother, she constantly clawed her own skin.

In interpreting your answers, don't concentrate on *meanings* at the expense of *themes*. What common chords unite the animals you've chosen? This is not exercise in logic: the wishes and fears beneath your symbol animals may be expressed subtly, even backward, and working them out demands more creativity than rationality. The person who chooses "tiger" as an animal because the tiger is allowed to be angry and no one can stop him and the person who wants to be a "lamb" because lambs are never angry are not opposites at all. To the contrary, they both need to work through the task of expressing anger—one of the eleven tasks discussed in Chapter 2.

Instead of asking what the test shows about your wishes and fears, a more useful question is where the *emotional action* is. The person who fears losing control and the person who craves freedom are dealing with the same issue but in different ways. They are both grappling with autonomy. The *area* of conflict and confusion is more important than the specific wishes and fears that define it. Try inverting your answers: imagine for a moment that the animals you chose as most desirable are actually the ones you least want to be, and vice versa. Play the game with an open mind and you may stumble over some very suggestive surprises.

The ultimate question, of course, is: why should the person who emerges from the Animal Test, who wants to be a dog but would hate to be a weasel, have your skin problem? Connecting your fantasy animals and your skin is a creative process, and I don't want to prescribe a rigid method for getting them. I would suggest being systematic, however.

In the first stage of the test, picking animals and saying why, don't even think about "what it all means." Just be spontaneous and honest with yourself. Wondering whether you're saying the right thing—self-editing—shuts down the creative process, as anyone who's struggled with "writer's block" can testify.

Once you've written down the raw material of your answers, look for themes—the ways in which positive choices and negative choices group around the same issues. What motifs recur?

Then try to connect these themes to the three fundamental needs for love, respect, and protection. How do these unresolved needs suggest emotional tasks? How might your skin be working to accomplish these tasks?

In actual practice, interpreting your answers will not be such a straightforward process. Possibly, as soon as you start thinking about your reasons for choosing "wolf," the need to express anger will come to mind, and you'll recognize this task in your other answers, too. Don't expect all your choices to focus on any one need or task. They may come from different corners of your complex personality, and thus arrange themselves in parallel, not converging, lines. Your answers will very possibly suggest three, even four tasks.

One question that some find fertile is: if you were any of these animals, what tasks *wouldn't* you face? The animals you'd like to be *have* what you wish for (at least in fantasy)—they've won the game just by being eagles or tigers. The ones you'd hate to be *can't* have what you wish—ants and cockroaches can't be loved, respected, or protected (at least in our human minds), so they needn't struggle for it.

In searching for needs and tasks in your answers, remember again that the key is not to be found in the animals themselves, but in their symbolic meaning to you, the "why" behind the choice. For example, one animal chosen by many people taking this test is the dog: this most familiar of beasts is popular both as the animal we'd most and least want to be. Depending on the reasons for the choice, "dog" can point toward any of the eleven tasks discussed in Chapter 2.

A dog chosen because he is "lovable, cuddly, and man's best friend," or rejected because "people forget to feed him" or because he's put in the doghouse, suggests concern with the task of "looking for love." If chosen because he can bark and bite and scare people, or rejected because he's kicked around—an underdog—the animal points to the task of "raging"—expressing anger. A person who'd like to be a watchdog, to keep people out of trouble, or who wouldn't want to be a dog that tears garbage apart and pees in the petunias, may be tangled up in the task of controlling "illegitimate" impulses and also using his skin as a policeman.

Here are some possible reasons for choosing or rejecting the dog, matched with the emotional tasks they suggest:

Why I'd most *like* to be a dog	Why I'd least *like* to be a dog	Related skin task
"lovable, cuddly, man's best friend"	"gets put in doghouse, ignored"	looking for love and protection (1)
"can bark and bite, scares people"	"underdog; kicked; not allowed to bite back"	raging (2)
"top dog"	"has to do what told; tied on leash; muzzled; locked in cage"	control (3)
"keeps people out of trouble; watchdog uninterested in sex (except when in heat)"	"tears garbage apart; pees in petunias; always humping everything"	sexual policeman (4)
"no memories, starts each day anew"	"once trained to do something, goes on forever"	rewriting history (5)
"you get kicked around, but they always feed you"	"gets kicked"	suffering for love (6)
"loyal; follows master anywhere; protects owner"	"imitates, follows owner everywhere; does stupidest things if told to"	loyalty (7)
"doesn't hide; face and tail tell everything; not devious like cats"	"can't hide anything; tail gives away feeling"	remembering and telling forbidden truths (8, 9)
"cute, cuddly puppy; dogs don't work or go to school; are children forever"	"too many puppies— not enough nipples; has to fight to survive"	freezing time (10)

Why I'd most *like to be a dog*	*Why I'd* least *like to be a dog*	*Related skin task*
"showdog—looks good but judges always take off points"	"can't maintain dignity; scratches, whimpers, drools, rolls on back"	telling world you're not perfect (11)

Note the examples (clearest in "loyalty" and "remembering") where the reasons given for most wanting and least wanting to be a dog are virtually the same. This should remind you that instead of simply asking what you're wishing and what you're fearing, it's more useful to ask yourself what issues are arousing both wishes and fears.

5

Why Now?

One thing just about all doctors do when they examine you is take a thorough history. They ask when the problem started, when it got worse, what similar difficulties you've had in the past. They often want to know about your health all the way back to childhood, and about your family's health as well.

It should be obvious that I'm vitally interested in history too. Already, you've been asked to look backward for insights into your inner self and its turmoil. The point is that any past event that still affects your life is not *just* history: it's alive in the present. The unresolved emotional tasks that complicate skin problems are chapters in your personal development that are relived, over and over.

Here we're going to attempt history on a grand scale: a reconstruction of the story of your life. No, I'm not suggesting that you take two years off and write your memoirs. More suited to our needs is something simpler: a Time Line like the one in high school history books that extends from 1400 to the present, with points indicating the discovery of America, the Revolutionary War, the invention of the steamboat, and World War II.

The Time Line is ideal for us for the same reason it was useful in high school history: it not only lets us see all the important events at once, but also reveals relationships between them. The Time Line in American History 2B suggested a pattern relating the invention of the cotton gin and the Civil War. Your own Time Line may show patterns in your history that have until now escaped your notice. When events are laid side by side, you may realize for the first time that your boils got much worse not long after your father left home. Or when your marriage deteriorated. Or that you first started flaking and scratching in the fourth grade, the same year that your family moved out to the suburbs and you had to change schools. The answer to "Why now?"—why your symptom developed the year, month, day it did—may point to where it came from, just as knowing why the Civil War started in 1860 will tell you much about the political, economic, and social forces that made it happen.

Take a very large sheet of paper—perhaps something like the oak-tag or stiff construction paper you used to make posters in grade school—and draw a horizontal line about one-fourth of the way down. The left end of the line is the moment of your conception, and the right end is the present, and in between are all the years of your life. Above the line, draw a vertical scale from one to one hundred, and on it a graph of your skin problem that begins with its first onset, rises when it got worse, and drops when it got better. One hundred on the scale is the worst it's ever been; zero is the best.

Below the line, list all the important events of your life, just under their appropriate years. Basically, these include everything that has made you the person you are.

This definitely means family events, such as the birth of siblings, people moving in or out of the house, deaths and major illness of anyone: parents, brothers, sisters, grandparents. If your mother or father was absent for a time, if a parent got a new job, or was fired or promoted, include it. Even less tangible events, like a shift in relationships—if you remember drawing closer to your brother around the time you were fifteen, put it in.

Add important events involving work and school: starting school, changing schools, honors, dishonors, and graduations. When did you start and leave each job? List all transfers, promotions, and shifts in duties. If particular events on the job stick in your mind—a fight or especially supportive relationship developing with a boss or coworker—put it in. Include big mo-

Time Line—Whole Life

(None of Main Skin Problems Yet)

Skin Rating: Worst 100 90 80 70 60 50 40 30 20 10 0 Best

	Feb 1959 Conception	Nov 1959 Birth	Jan '60	Jan '61	Jan '62
Skin & Medical			Colicky baby	Cradle cap (mild) Diaper rash (bad)	"Sensitive skin" unclear what that really means
Family & Marriage	Mother very morning-sick	Brother (age 3) had weird rash Sister (age 6) wetting bed	Hard to get a straight story but sounds like mother spent 3–6 months in major postpartum depression Mother's mother (MGM) came to stay—very helpful but made everyone edgy Brother broke arm—whole family *still* feels guilty	Brother used to honk horn & wake me up Sister suggested trading me for a puppy	Finally sleeping through the night Mother's mother moved out Father around more again
School & Work	Job change—Father traveled much more				
Sex		Mother hints Father also withdrew sexually at this point			
Other Ideas, Hunches, Hearsay	Father had sworn "no more kids, they are draining the life out of us"	I was very purple, wrinkled but bright-eyed at birth— Father out of town	Delivery difficult— mother said "you almost killed me"	Slow to walk and talk— parents seemed unnecessarily worried according to Aunt Ellen "A good eater" but mother reports this in tone of voice that doesn't make it sound good	

Skin Rating

Best — 80 70 60 50 40 30 20 10 0

	March	April	May	June	July	Aug	Sept	Oct	Nov	Dec	Jan	Feb	March	April
Skin & Medical			Skin seemed sensitive no visible problem				A bit of irritation/creme cured it			Insomnia	Back Spasms	Irritation/creme not working		*First serious skin eruption*
Family & Marriage						Wife has urinary tract infection		Wife withdrawn & surly (44–50)		Wife away: trial separation (65–75)			Filed for divorce (73–90)	
School Work		Made up of new company after merger (29-15)			National award (28-5)			Boss a pain (23-10)				New division head named (29-50)		
Sex					Wife seemed strange sexually (39-75)			Sex now just a memory (39-75)						
Other		Beat Fred at tennis for first time	Car trouble / Cat ran away "our child"	Cut back on socializing (18-5)		Car trouble		Moved to new house (31-10)(25-10)	Mother-in-law running wild (29-50)	Christmas (rough) (12-20)		Car finally fixed	House needs new roof	

First number: Holmes & Rahe rating
Second number: Your own rating

ments in athletics and turning points in friendships. Things that disappointed you by not happening are as real as things that did happen: don't forget to put in the time you didn't make the team.

Sexual events may be particularly important; jot down all the milestones. Going way back, note when you first discovered the difference between little boys and little girls, when you first played "doctor," when you first masturbated, began to menstruate. Include your first boyfriend or girlfriend, first kiss, petting, intercourse. Any event that stands out in your sexual life deserves to be noted just because you remember it: starts and ends of significant relationships, fights, high points, even orgasms you'll never forget. (Note: here and throughout this exercise, don't skip topics that make you uncomfortable—these may be the most important. If you wish, use a code on the Time Line to ensure secrecy.) Childbirth and abortion are important parts of your sexual history.

Your medical history is highly relevant. Place in its appropriate spot any significant illnesses you've suffered, any operations or major medical procedures. Needless to say, put in everything dermatological.

If there's *anything* that impresses you with its emotional impact, give it space on the Time Line—pets, family fights, trips and travels, periods when you were depressed and didn't know why, any significant change or turning point. The rule is: if it seems important, it *is* important.

This exercise is not the work of an afternoon. It's a personal research project you will have to live with for weeks, perhaps months. In my experience, many people get impressive results quite quickly—in a few hours, they've gotten down the basics, perhaps twelve of the most important events of their lives. After that, there's often a long period where they return to the project from time to time, adding important events as they come to mind, touching up, filling in, and refining the Time Line.

Try posting the Time Line on your bedroom or bathroom wall, so you can add details as they occur to you. Once you get your mind on the proper wavelength, information and memories gradually percolate and drift up to the surface. You'll probably discover a wealth of material that was in "inactive storage"—accessible to your memory, but not *immediately* accessible. As you sift through your memory bank, the most important things will emerge.

How can you discover what events, what needs and fears and emotional tasks, inhabit the deep parts of your mind, where today, yesterday, and infancy sit side by side? It is here that your Time Line can yield the fullest dividends. Pressing relentlessly to reconstruct these years that are both dim and distant and vibrantly alive, you are seeking to find out what makes you who you really are.

Constructing your Time Line is a lengthy task, but one that will reward you with insights all along the way, and once you've gotten the first ten or so pivotal life events down, you've made a significant start. As you search for and wait for more details to bubble up to the surface, relax: you're your own biographer here, but you needn't worry about the scrupulous standards of objective accuracy that bind most biographers—our goal is *psychological* reality. If you remember that your mother was out of town for six months when you were five years old, and she tells you that in fact she took a two-week trip to Baltimore when you were seven, your version is the "right" one for your purposes. As a small child, you experienced her loss as prolonged: the distortions of memory are a lie that tells the truth.

Help from relatives may be invaluable when you're trying to reconstruct early events, which deserve particular attention if your skin problem began when you were young. Find out what you can about the big moments of those years, tapping the memories of your parents, older brothers and sisters, and uncles and aunts. If you were born with a skin problem, find out what was happening in your family during the preceding year—this may have influenced the prenatal environment in which you developed.

The Time Line is a wide-angle panorama that portrays your whole life at once. Later I'll show you how to move in for a close-up of a critical period.

Now let's look at some striking research that will help us get maximum benefit from the Time Line.

If you've picked up a magazine or newspaper or turned on the TV news in recent years, you've no doubt heard all about "stress," and the way that emotional experiences can affect your body profoundly enough to make you ill. Studies have linked diseases including heart attack, ulcer, and infection to stress. If (for genetic or unknown reasons) your skin is your body's weakest link, it is here that emotional turmoil is likely to take its toll.

But what causes stress, exactly? There's a general answer, which is useful, and a more personal, psychological answer that will be much more useful. According to psychiatrists Thomas Holmes and Richard Rahe, there are certain events, like many on your Time Line, that cause stress to everyone. Holmes and Rahe call them "life changes." They developed a scale that lists major life-change events and approximates how much stress each would cause the average person.

Their chart covers the gamut of human experience. The most stressful change is the death of a spouse; divorce is not far behind. No one would argue with the impact of these losses on anyone. But some other stress sources may surprise you. "Changing to a different line of work" is often a change for the better. We usually think of "outstanding personal achievement" as a cause for celebration. Yet Drs. Holmes and Rahe rate it as stressful as "in-law troubles."[1]

The essential ingredient all these events share is change. Any change, good or bad, forces your mind—and your body—to adapt. If too much is demanded in too little time, your body's adaptation energy is exhausted. Psychologically, all change involves loss—a promotion at work, for example, means the loss of familiar duties, roles, and relationships. And loss means emotional and physical wear and tear.

The effects of stress and loss are *cumulative*. In a series of studies, Drs. Holmes and Rahe asked subjects from different cultures and walks of life to score and total up all their life changes from the past year. They found (with surprising uniformity, considering the diversity of the people they studied) that those with a score greater than 300 in one year had an 80 percent chance of falling ill. When the score fell into the 200–299 range, the odds for illness were 50 percent. People who tallied 150 to 200 points had a 37 percent risk of health problems.[2]

Can you see such a pattern behind your skin disorder? Examine the section of your Time Line that extends a year before your symptom developed, note events in the Holmes-Rahe table of life changes, and add up your score. Do the same tabulation for years preceding major flare-ups. You may want to compare these scores with "normal" one-year periods of your life.

This is just the beginning, however. Drs. Holmes and Rahe studied the way people respond to stressful events *on average*. You are unique; what's important—here's a notion we'll return to time and again—is the meaning of these events in *your* mind, and their effect on *your* body.

To take a familiar example, day-to-day irritations, like parking problems and fights with the boss, are also stressful. Yet individual reactions differ enormously. Consider two men in the same traffic jam. One is fuming, tapping his fingers, constantly rechecking his watch and ruminating over time lost. The other has resigned himself to waiting as an unattractive but inevitable feature of city life: he's using the time to mull over a work-related problem, while he listens to music on his tape deck. On the same highway—perhaps in the same car—one man is under stress, the other is not.

By the same token, your neighbor's divorce may be very different from your divorce, and the 73 points assigned to this life-change event on the Holmes-Rahe scale may be inappropriate to both (even though it is accurate for the average). "Troubles with boss" may have one meaning to a person who has difficulty dealing with authority, and an entirely different one for another who has achieved a philosophical attitude toward the compromises we must make to earn a living. To the first, such troubles "cost" far more than the 23 stress points assigned by the Holmes-Rahe scale; to the second, far less.

To personalize your stress score, go back to your Time Line and reconsider the years before your skin problem started and worsened significantly. List again the significant changes that took place. Refer to the Holmes-Rahe chart again, but this time adjust its point values up or down depending on *what each event actually meant to you.*

Are these cumulative scores significantly different from your first totals? Can you see a pattern? Some people rate their own

LIFE EVENT	NUMBER OF OCCURRENCES	SCALE VALUE	YOUR SCORE
Death of spouse		100	
Divorce		73	
Marital separation from mate		65	
Detention in jail or other institution		63	
Death of a close family member		63	
Major personal injury or illness		53	
Marriage		50	
Being fired at work		47	
Marital reconciliation with mate		45	
Retirement from work		45	
Major change in the health or behavior of a family member		44	
Pregnancy		40	
Sexual difficulties		39	
Gaining a new family member (e.g., through birth, adoption, oldster moving in, etc.)		39	
Major business readjustment (e.g., merger, reorganization, bankruptcy, etc.)		39	
Major change in financial state (e.g., a lot worse off or a lot better off than usual)		38	
Death of a close friend		37	
Changing to a different line of work		36	
Major change in the number of arguments with spouse (e.g., either a lot more or a lot less than usual regarding child-rearing, personal habits, etc.)		35	
Taking on a mortgage greater than $10,000 (e.g., purchasing a house, business, etc.)		31	
Foreclosure on a mortgage or loan		30	
Major change in responsibilities at work (e.g., promotion, demotion, lateral transfer)		29	
Son or daughter leaving home (e.g., marriage, attending college, etc.)		29	
In-law troubles		29	
Outstanding personal achievement		28	
Wife beginning or ceasing work outside the home		26	
Beginning or ceasing formal schooling		26	

LIFE EVENT	NUMBER OF OCCURRENCES	SCALE VALUE	YOUR SCORE
Major change in living conditions (e.g., building a new house, remodeling, deterioration of house or neighborhood)		25	
Revision of personal habits (dress, manners, associations, etc.)		24	
Troubles with boss		23	
Major change in working hours or conditions		20	
Change in residence		20	
Changing to a new school		20	
Major change in usual type and/or amount of recreation		19	
Major change in church activities (e.g., a lot more or a lot less than usual)		19	
Major change in social activities (e.g., clubs, dancing, movies, visiting, etc.)		18	
Taking on a mortgage or loan less than $10,000 (e.g., purchasing a car, TV, freezer, etc.)		17	
Major change in sleeping habits (a lot more or a lot less sleep, or change in part of day when asleep)		16	
Major change in number of family get-togethers (e.g., a lot more or a lot less than usual)		15	
Major change in eating habits (a lot more or a lot less food intake, or very different meal hours or surroundings)		15	
Vacation		13	
Christmas		12	
Minor violations of the law (e.g., traffic tickets, jaywalking, disturbing the peace, etc.)		11	
This is your total life change score for the past year			

SOURCE: *The Schedule of Recent Experience (SRE)*, © 1976 by Thomas H. Holmes, M.D.

reactions consistently less intense than the average, which raises some useful questions. Are they out of touch with their feelings? Do they deny or suppress their emotions more than most people? Do you rate *certain* events higher in stress than Holmes and Rahe—"changes for the better" like promotions, for example, or relationship ups and downs? If so, you may have unearthed a valuable clue to your needs, fears, and emotional tasks.[3]

The question is: where does your heightened reaction come from? Why is a business failure, say, distressing but surmountable for Robert G., but devastating for Horace T.? At every moment, in every situation, you react with a personality that comes in part from your genetic heritage, but for the most part has been shaped and molded by the experiences you've accumulated throughout your life.

To put it simply, your earlier years are not just past history. The emotionally vibrant events with which you never came fully to terms are alive and active in your here-and-now life, vulnerable and sensitive, an emotional Achilles heel. All the losses, frustrations, and confrontations of your life are connected like the links of a chain: if you rattle one, all the others will rattle.

When you feel you're overreacting to an apparently unimportant event, it's because you're *also* responding to all the earlier events that the experience brings to mind—not one link in the chain, but a dozen. *The heart does not overreact.* This will become clear as you understand the past events that survive, alive and kicking, in the parts of yourself that escape the laws of time.

For example, suppose a major skin flare-up appears to have been triggered by the breakup of a casual relationship—a rejection by someone who didn't mean very much to you. Why the devastating effect on your skin? An introspective look backward may reveal that loss and rejection loom large in your life story. Look back far enough, and you may find a similar loss in the childhood days when you were most needy and vulnerable—the prolonged absence of a parent, or a pronounced emotional withdrawal—that *sensitized* you to the losses you would experience ten, twenty, forty years later.

To use an analogy, a person who is allergic to bee venom can suffer a violent reaction, even die, when stung. Not the first time, but after one or more stings have created a sensitivity. If such a reaction occurs, it is misleading to say that the "trigger" was the sting that occurred two minutes earlier, ignoring the earlier ones that made him sensitive. To understand his vulnerability, you must look back over the years: the stings of ten, even twenty years ago are still alive in the antibodies that circulate in his bloodstream.

In reconstructing the events that inhabit the deep parts of your mind (where today, yesterday, and infancy sit side by side), your Time Line yields its fullest dividends. Pressing to recapture those early years that are both dim and distant and vibrantly alive, you are finding out what makes you who you really are. As you fill out your Time Line with all the significant events that have remained in your memory, be alert for motifs and patterns. Many of these events have stuck with you because they are connected to your wishes and fears. Your Time Line, then, is a map of emotional hot spots: the prominence of events having to do with anger, or rejection, or loss, or guilt, may lead to a new understanding of emotional tasks that keep your skin disease hard at work.

One of my genital herpes patients, for example, noted how childhood events involving sexuality stood out on her Time Line. She recalled her parents' dismay and her own shame when they caught her and a little neighbor boy "playing doctor." The onset of menstruation was a moment of anxiety, again reinforced by parental reaction. As her memories of those years come clear, she came to appreciate how her early years had sensitized her to the whole issue of sex—how her parents' discomfort had silently taught the lesson that sex was an anxious business.

Her herpes, then, had stirred up a feeling of uneasiness that had been planted long before in her mind. Her genitals were now truly defective and unclean—as she had always suspected: herpes, for her, was more than a physical illness, the focus of fears and anxieties with roots in the long-ago. Realizing the connection between her troubled sexual feelings and her herpes anxiety was extremely comforting: the distress now *made sense*—given the logic of her own psychology, she wasn't crazy to feel as bad as she did. She could begin to bring these feelings out into the light of day, and release herself from their grip.

Why was the remembered shame and anxiety my patient experienced when discovered "playing doctor" important? This event, in itself, didn't *shape* her attitudes toward sex. But it dramatically displays the forces of her upbringing that molded her personality, and the uneasiness within that had already taken hold. Remembered moments like this are flashes of insight that reveal what life was really like in critically formative years—and what it is like, still, in the timeless reaches of your mind. Her recollection *points* to sexuality as an unanswered question mixed up in her troubled skin.

The Time Line and the understanding of emotional tasks you've derived from other exercises complement each other. If you've come to feel that the expression of anger and the quest for control, for example, are involved in your skin problem, devote special attention to Time Line events that got you angry and where you felt your freedom was threatened or trampled—a history of anger and autonomy. Seemingly trivial details may start to fall into place—how your mother or sister insisted on walking you to school while all the other kids were allowed to make it on their own; or how you burned impotently when your sixth-grade teacher exposed you to public humiliation because you couldn't master fractions. Gradually, you may work back and forth between details and your emerging sense of the whole, as many historical researchers do: as patterns emerge, they guide you to where it will be most profitable to look.

To put it most simply, the Time Line is also another way to focus in on the question of the last chapter: Why you? Everyone has the same basic needs and deals with the same emotional tasks—why did these particular needs and tasks come to be mixed up with your physical health? As we discussed earlier, many physical symptoms are ways of reliving the emotional past, valiant, doomed attempts to solve the same problem over and over. "Those who are ignorant of history are doomed to repeat it" is as true in psychology as in politics. In becoming less ignorant of your history, you may learn to unearth the buried past and its feelings, and release your skin from its painful grip.

THE MICRO TIME LINE

"Why now?" has another meaning for skin sufferers. Why did I have to have a hives outbreak today? Why is my eczema so much worse *this week* than it was last week? Why am I suddenly starting to itch? The same process that links emotional turmoil to illness operates on a small scale in day-to-day, week-to-week ups and downs of your symptom. Most of my patients find that tun-

The Griesemer Index:
How Often Emotions Trigger Skin Problems

Diagnosis	Percentage of diagnoses emotionally triggered	Biologic incubation interval between stress and start of problem
Profuse sweating	100	Seconds
Severe scratching	98	Seconds
Focused itching	98	Days to 2 weeks
Specific hair loss	96	2 weeks
Warts, multiple spreading	95	Days
Rosacea	94	2 days
Itching	86	Seconds
Lichen planus	82	Days to 2 weeks
Hand eczema (dyshidrosis)	76	2 days for vesicles
Atopic eczema	70	Seconds for itching
Self-inflicted wounds	69	Seconds
Hives	68	Minutes
Psoriasis	62	Days to 2 weeks
Traumatic eczema	56	Seconds
All eczema except contact	56	Days
Acne	55	2 days for tender red papules
Diffuse hair loss	55	2–3 weeks
Nummular eczema	52	Days
Seborrheic eczema	41	Days to 2 weeks
Herpes: oral, genital, zoster	36	Days
Vitiligo	33	2–3 weeks
Nail dystrophy	29	2–3 weeks
Pyoderma	29	Days
Bacterial infections	29	Days
Cysts	27	2–3 weeks
Contact eczema	15	2 days
Fungus infections	9	Days to 2 weeks
Keratoses	0	—
Basal cell cancer	0	—
Nevi	0	—

NOTE: These figures are quite conservative but useful for comparisons. (T. G.)

Adapted from Robert D. Griesemer, M.D., Assistant Clinical Professor of Dermatology, Harvard Medical School ing in to these variations helps them get a good handle on the problems under their skin: patterns are easier to see than the year-long contours of the Time Line.

Over the course of a year, dermatologist Robert E. Griese-mer spent a few minutes talking to each of his patients about his or her life. He asked what upsets had occurred in the days or weeks preceding the flare-up that brought the patient in for treatment. Had there been quarrels at home? Pressure at school or on the job? With many skin conditions, a clear connection was evident in a high percentage of cases.

Fifty-six percent of certain eczemas were apparently triggered by emotional upset, for example, and 62 percent of psoriasis flareups. Emotions had a triggering role in nearly all cases of severe scratching, hyperhidrosis (excessive sweating), alopecia areata (hair loss), and rosacea. Emotional stress surely did not cause viral problems, but it could set them off: the link was evident in 36 percent of outbreaks of herpes simplex (cold sores and genital herpes) and 95 percent of multiple spreading warts.[4]

If anything, Dr. Griesemer's research *underestimated* the importance of emotional triggers. His inquiries were modest by psychological standards: he did not probe problems in depth, and conspicuously avoided questions about sex—clearly an important area. Many people are simply unaware of what's causing them distress, particularly when besieged by both physical and emotional problems. Many of Dr. Griesemer's patients may not have noticed the upsetting circumstances that preceded their flare-ups, and others may simply not have wanted to talk about them.

Are emotional triggers a critical factor in your skin condition? Your Time Line gives important clues if it reveals memorably upsetting events in the year before its onset and major turns for the worse. The pattern may come clearer, however, with a variation: the Micro Time Line.

If the Time Line is a telescope enabling you to look back over your life with a new appreciation of its distant contours, the Micro Time Line is a microscope to examine small patches of time in detail. Your skin's daily ups and downs are little echoes of major flare-ups and remissions, and may mirror their connection to your emotional life.

SAMPLE MICRO TIME LINE

		1 2 3 4 5 6 7 8 9 10 11 12 13 14 15 16 17 18 19 20 21 22 23 24 25
Worst	100	
	90	
	80	
	70	
	60	
Amount	50	
of	40	
Irritation	30	
	20	
	10	
Best	0	

Event	1 2 3 4 5 6 7 8 9 10 11 12 13 14 15 16 17 18 19 20 21 22 23 24 25
Time	7:30 a.m.　　　　　　9 a.m.　　　　　　12–1 p.m.　　2:30 p.m.

1. Woke up
2. Back hurt
3. Turned on radio
4. Wife grumpy—wonder if I did something
5. Looked in mirror—what a mess
6. Shower—saw more bad skin
7. Brushed teeth, toilet, hair combed
8. Clothes didn't look right as dressing
9. Breakfast tasty
10. Car started in spite of cold
11. Traffic moderate
12. Good music on radio
13. News less ridiculous than usual
14. Receptionist smiled at work
15. Boss superficially warm but underlying condescension
16. Wave of self-doubt
17. Obsessing about report
18. Secretary tries to be nice
19. Wondering why get stuck with her
20. Bump knee—pissed
21. Lunch with Charlie—he's an "up"
22. Fish was good
23. Rush back to office—resent it
24. Too many phone calls
25. Everyone wants miracles

*Over the micro time interval, not worst & best ever.

On another piece of paper (smaller than the Time Line poster) chart the variations in your skin condition for several days, possibly a week—long enough, in any case, for it to get better and worse (even minimally) three or four times. Beneath the line, record everything else that's happening in your life—good times and bad times; life within the family; deadline pressures and minor triumphs and setbacks at the office. Remember to include the good with the bad, and to leave nothing out because it seems trivial. If you were upset by a news item, an overheard remark, or a soap-opera tragedy; if you felt depressed because it was rainy or cheerful because you saw the first crocus of spring, be sure to record it.

When looking for patterns, don't be confused if emotional events and skin changes are separated by a time lag of a few days or longer. Dr. Griesemer found such "incubation periods" to be common. There was a lapse of several days between apparent trigger and outbreak of eczema, for example, and as long as two weeks for fungus and bacterial infections; episodes of hyperhidrosis and neurotic excoriation, on the other hand, followed triggering stress in seconds.

Many of my patients have found this exercise instructive simply because they never before were conscious that their skin problems changed so noticeably from hour to hour and day to day. From this insight it was a short step to tuning in to particular events that seemed to make the problem better, or worse.

The connections between life and skin may be very obvious, as demonstrated by the skin patients who were unwitting participants—victims may be a better word—in a cruel experiment performed by Australian army doctors just after World War II. One, who had been a dentist in civilian life but was unable to practice his profession in the army, had severe eczema on his hands. When he was told by his superiors that his retirement from the army was imminent, his hands improved dramatically. Then the doctors had him informed that instead of retirement, he could look forward to a transfer to the infantry: within four and a half hours, his eczema returned in force.[5]

The patterns you'll find will probably be more subtle. As with the Time Line exercise, you may get essential insights by discovering *what kind of* irritation, anxiety, upset, or stress gives your skin grief. Certain of my patients with severe recurrent genital herpes, for example, have learned to distinguish between what they call "garden-variety stress" and "herpes stress." "Some weeks, my life is a zoo," one patient told me. "Everything is a rush and I'm just climbing the walls. But I know I'm not going to have a herpes outbreak. No way. It's not the kind of stress that gives me a recurrence. Other days are less hectic, but I know my herpes will act up because what's happening is the things that trigger outbreaks. That's herpes stress."

In exactly the same way, you have your own vulnerability to "hives stress" or "ichthyosis stress." Getting to recognize which of life's ups, downs, and hassles pushes the psychological button to make your skin suffer, you'll find another avenue to understanding the mind-body wiring behind the scenes.

6

The Self-Sabotage Test

The value of last chapter's Time Line and Micro Time Line is most clear when they reveal parallel patterns linking life and skin. If setbacks, tensions, and stress are followed by outbreaks and flare-ups, you'll see it in your Time Lines.

But things aren't always this simple and logical. Were you frustrated to find no apparent connection between stress and symptoms? Did it seem that, if anything, your skin was *better* in hectic, deadline crunching weeks; that it stayed clear through domestic turmoil and office shakeups, only to give you grief when every other part of your life was under control, and all your other systems "go"? If so, you're not some kind of freak. There's logic here too, only it requires a bit more effort to understand, and a different kind of test to identify.

To return to a cardinal principle, what matters to your health is less what happens out there in the world than its *translation* by your mind and its experience by your body. And what causes skin troubles for you is not some universal stress formula but your own personal combination of events and reactions to them that adds up to "shingles stress," "eczema stress," "psoriasis stress," or whatever.

History illustrates this principle. Time and again, physicians have found that the extreme stress of war causes no increase in skin ailments—not for soldiers in battle, civilians under siege, or prisoners of war.[1] Northern Ireland's perpetual conflict makes it a living stress laboratory, to take a modern example. Civil unrest, occupation, terrorist bombs—by any standards, a most unsettling environment. A study there found *some* cases where traumatic events apparently triggered skin symptoms (a twenty-one-year old man, for example, developed seborrheic eczema two days after being injured by a bomb). But in general, researchers have seen no significant rise in skin disease, regardless of the level of stress.[2] By and large, people caught up in the nightmare of history don't suffer the physical symptoms of those enmeshed in their own emotional turmoil.

Even in the midst of mass murder—in the concentration camps of Nazi Germany—stress remains resolutely personal. Dr. Jacob Shannon of Hadassah Medical Center in Israel surveyed camp survivors with skin problems and found that some had indeed developed them, particularly eczema, dry skin, hives, and psoriasis, while imprisoned. But the picture was different with a second group. These suffered no skin symptoms despite the humiliation, privation, and brutality that marked life in the camps. Their symptoms—typically itching and neurodermatitis—appeared shortly *after their release*. What was the logic here?

Dr. Shannon hypothesized two categories of symptoms. Those with an obvious connection to real-life difficulties he called *stress-ogenic*—they were generated by the pain and hardship of camp life. The second group he called *conflictogenic*—the source of illness here was an inner conflict that the outer stress aroused.

In detailed psychological interviews, differences between the groups became clear. The stressogenic people could talk freely about their camp experiences, while the conflictogenic ones could not—they acted as if a buried sense of guilt kept them silent. Indeed, while the stressogenic patients apparently thought of themselves as victims, the conflictogenic group seemed to feel they were guilty for things that had happened in the camps.

Such reactions, while obviously illogical, are far from rare. Guilt and rage are often the lasting legacy of degradation and abuse. The "crime" may be the failure to save the life of a loved one or dear friend—even though the self-scourging "criminal" was himself absolutely powerless. Or just surviving when so many others perished.

The conflictogenic symptoms that first appeared after release from the camps continued to follow the same pattern in later years, Dr. Shannon discovered. While life was hard, these patients had no trouble with their skin; it only flared up when times were easy. It seemed that their skin had the role of *punishing* them, but only when life failed to supply enough hard knocks—only then did it have to remind them of what had happened, and what they had done.[3]

This paradoxical pattern—skin gets bad when life is good—isn't limited to extreme cases. If "self-punishment" sounds too harsh, think of it as "self-sabotage," a widespread phenomenon that has received well-deserved attention in recent years, usually linked with so-called "fear of success." Many people strive for success on one hand, but fear and flee it on the other. "Success," after all, can mean guilt at besting a parent's achievements, or anxiety at becoming a conspicuous target for the envy of others. It means giving up familiar roles and comfortable camaraderie for new, taxing duties and a position that frequently alienates old friends and coworkers. Consequently, we may *sabotage* our own best efforts—often unconsciously. We clutch in crisis, forget important things, fall short of our potential, to avoid the perils of the success we consciously want.

The skin can play a role in this flight from success, as you know if you've ever had a severe attack of whatever ails you on the eve of a critical meeting. But self-sabotage can also satisfy any number of other emotional needs.

Many of us are familiar with the almost superstitious fear that we must "pay dues" in one form or another, that if things go too well, fate will strike us down. The suggestion that you must suffer to be saved is deeply woven into some religions, along with the mirror notion that good fortune now means trouble later: a rich man, it is said, will find it hard to enter heaven. So self-sabotage can be a kind of self-protection; and a skin condition, sensitive and responsive to emotional needs, can step in when life itself isn't giving enough hard knocks. When other troubles take over this work—a discord at home or trouble with the car—the skin is free to get better.

The need to temper good fortune with suffering may be rooted in personal history. One of my patients recalled his high school years as a dramatic turning point in his life. He was coming very much into his own as a young man at that time: active, popular, successful at school. Then the roof fell in: his parents divorced, his mother became psychotic and had to be hospitalized. Later in life, he was dogged by a fear of being too happy and doing too well. Would good fortune bring about another catastrophe?

More generally, self-sabotage can serve the emotional tasks I talked about earlier. When the lesson has been learned that pain comes hand in hand with love ("the skin suffers for love"), a harsh form of self-sabotage is an unfailing source of that pain.

Less dramatically, the skin's self-sabotage can ensure loyalty to a long-suffering parent. I'm talking of the mother or father who always tuned in to the dark side of any situation—a person who would pause ominously when asked "How are you?" and who couldn't watch a baseball game without clucking severely about how the players were overpaid. In childhood, the only way to stay close to such a parent might have been to share his or her gloomy visions, to nod in sympathy at the moronity of the commercials that constantly interrupted the evening movie and to refrain from enthusiasm over the movie itself. Once learned, this style can continue into adulthood, and a skin condition that acts up when life has nothing else sufficiently negative to offer can be a lifelong way of agreeing that it's a cruel world.

A child who grew up with parents who came through admirably when he was sick or suffered a setback but tended to ignore him when all went well may have learned the lesson that at least a little bit of trouble is a requirement for proper caring ("the skin seeks love and protection"). His skin condition may stand forever on the sidelines, ready to go into the game when nothing else is providing the quota of trouble.

The important point is that your skin symptom is one way, *but not the only way*, to accomplish emotional tasks through self-sabotage. If you have a sore throat, you don't need your eczema to keep you home from work and allow you the privilege of childlike incapacity. Your skin symptom is only one real-life difficulty that can get you sympathy or protection or help you maintain control over others. Pain and trouble of any kind reminds the world you're not perfect. Skin symptoms themselves can alternate like partners in a tag-team wrestling match. One patient of mine had acne outbreaks only when he didn't have herpes outbreaks: each made him feel an unlovable loser, unable to strive for relationship or career goals.

The pattern here is very different from stress-symptom link I talked about in Chapter 5. Here they aren't cause and effect but two members of the same team: when life is difficult, your skin symptom can take a rest; it's more likely to flare up when times are easy. You can see if this process is operating for you by going back to your time lines and applying the Self-Sabotage Test.

First, look at your big Time Line again, this time asking different questions. Did anything strikingly *good* happen just before your skin condition appeared or flared up? Did anything *bad* happen any time before it improved? You also want to apply the Self-Sabotage Test to your Micro Time Line. To do this properly you'll have to extend it for several weeks: keep careful note of how your skin gets better and worse from day to day, and alongside keep tabs on whatever is happening—*good and bad*—in your life. Remember the incubation periods that Dr. Griesemer noted, and be alert for skin-condition changes that follow a few days to two weeks after life events. If you find that keeping a journal comes more naturally, simply record in detail the events of each day, and the condition of your skin.

The pattern to look for, again, is where other setbacks and misfortunes—quarrels, business difficulties, traffic jams—allow your skin to improve. In particular, keep a close eye on what happens to your skin when you get sick with (or recover from) unrelated health problems. Many people find that when other illnesses take over the task of paying dues, their skin gets better.

If you see a self-sabotage pattern, follow your big Time Line back into your early history for events that might have established it: times, for example, when things were "too good" and then were swiftly undercut by misfortune; situations that taught you the dangers of aiming high and making it. A positive Self-Sabotage Test may open up a new perspective on the emotional tasks that lie beneath your troubled skin, and how your symptoms satisfy these tasks.

Looking at the data of your life from a number of perspectives is complicated work. What you are doing here is a kind of research. Like the investigators whose work I've cited, you're taking on the subtlety and complexity of human experience, and searching for the truth beneath the surface. To make it all the more exciting, the subject of your study is yourself, and the surface is your troubled skin.

7

Why There?
Mapping Trouble Spots

Introducing the Animal Test in Chapter 4, I talked about how the inner self often communicates best through symbols—objects invested with emotion and meaning. (The deer is more than just a shy animal—it seems like shyness come to life: the *symbol* of shyness.) Such symbols are common in art, poetry, and everyday figures of speech.

We live with and through our bodies, and in them we find symbols for the whole range of human experience. Body parts become identified with what they do, embodying abstractions like deceit ("giving lip service") and devotion ("I only have eyes for you"). A person who refuses to be moved from the spot, intellectually or emotionally, is "putting her foot down." Body symbols are embedded in the language of daily life: we manipulate and control objects with our hands, so there's poetic logic in a word denoting how we *handle* ourselves, others, our jobs, our lives.

Through body symptoms, the inner self expresses its needs, wishes, and fears. These are often pragmatic if misguided efforts to accomplish emotional tasks, like the woman whose outbreak of genital herpes literally resolved her "should I or shouldn't I?" sexual conflict. But symptoms may also be *symbolic* expressions of these needs and tasks. The early literature of psychiatry is filled with cases of "hysterical conversion"—men and women who became blind, deaf, even paralyzed, for no physical reason. Their eyes, ears, and whatever were in perfect working order, but ceased to function normally in order to express emotional conflict in an extreme form of body language. Here the location of the problem was an essential part of the message—like the noun in a sentence. The woman who became blind after catching a glimpse of a parent's infidelity—an expression of her shock and horror at what she'd seen—was not going to become deaf instead.

A similar kind of symbolism may be less dramatic: a persistent ache in the upper back, for example, might express the feeling that one is "carrying the world on one's shoulders" and needs relief. There may be similar revealing logic in the place where your skin symptom chooses to appear or intensify: the answer to "why there?" is often a key phrase in the message your skin is struggling to convey.

The question sometimes seems pointless: your contact dermatitis developed *there*, on your hands, because they were in contact with a noxious chemical. A rash developed *there*, on your feet, because they provided a warm, moist climate ideal for a fungus or irritation. Certain skin diseases have a predilection for certain parts of the body—acne is most likely on the face or back, for example. Even here, however, asking "why there?" may clue you in to your symptom's hurting and staying power: what keeps it holding on.

To ask "why there?" profitably, you need an open mind willing to make creative connections. Why did your eczema choose to appear around your eyes? What difference does it make to you that your arms are afflicted with hives, rather than your legs? The physical scene of the dermatological crime may point, via metaphor, to where the action is emotionally.

One of my patients, for example, was driven by an uncontrollable urge to scratch her arms, a nightly scourge (*excoriation* is the medical term) that left them swollen and bleeding. In therapy, it became clear that many of Maggie D.'s problems involved her feelings about her mother, who seemed loving but was actually a constricting, manipulative person. Not only wasn't Maggie able to express the anger she felt at her mother's manipulations, she felt intensely guilty over the fact that she'd been angry at all.

That her arms were the target of Maggie's self-attacks was not accidental. These are the classic instruments of aggression as well as affection. Unable to strike out at her mother in anger, she attacked the instrument with which she *would* strike out. In scratching her arms, she was metaphorically expressing her anger—and also punishing herself for it.

Note that I used the word "metaphorically" to describe how Maggie's skin was expressing itself. A metaphor usually means a figure of speech, the kind of thing that poets use to convey complex emotions in concrete form. In Shakespeare's play, "How sharper than a serpent's tooth it is to have a thankless child!" evokes King Lear's lacerating sense of his daughter's betrayal better than paragraphs of logical analysis ever could. Maggie's inner self was perhaps speaking like a poet in the language of emotions, with a complex, evocative metaphor: "I'm striking out and keeping myself from striking out and punishing myself for even thinking of striking out." To clarify the point, let's look at two specific ways in which "why there?" may link physical symptom and emotional action: metaphors before the fact and after the fact.

When it is a *metaphor before the fact*, the place where the skin symptom appears is integral to its meaning. Like hysterical blindness, there would be no point in its appearing elsewhere. The dermatologists Obermeyer, Wittkower, and Edgell, pioneers in the field of emotions and skin, describe one young woman who was kissed against her will by a suitor she found repugnant. The next day, she developed a skin irritation around her mouth —an expression, in skin language, of how she felt about the kiss!

They describe another patient who developed a rash on a single finger—one she used in sexual play—after she began a guilt-ridden extramarital affair.[1] Here the affliction was a physical expression of her guilt. On a more "innocent" part of her anatomy that had not been involved in the misdeed, the message of the symptom would have been lost.

In these cases, there was a literal connection between the body part, the actual event, and the symptom that followed. A metaphor before the fact may arise from a more figurative connection. The same authors describe a man who developed a rash on his navel shortly after the death of his mother. This was the point where he was "cut off" from his mother at birth, and it was at this part of his body that he metaphorically expressed his sense of loss now.

When a skin symptom happened where it happened because of physical factors—irritating contact, for example—"why there?" won't tell you its psychological underpinnings. But it may help you to understand the emotional resonance that makes it particularly upsetting and gives it power to hang on. Once established, a symptom can become a *metaphor after the fact:* it gathers strength from the meaning of the afflicted body part.

The power of metaphor after the fact is clear in the case of herpes. Biologically, oral and genital herpes are similar. They are caused by viruses so nearly alike that it takes an electron microscope to distinguish between them. In fact, 20 percent of genital herpes is caused by the virus that usually causes oral herpes. Psychologically, however, these are very different disorders: oral herpes is generally dismissed as the nuisance of "cold sores," while the latter can become the focus of devastating emotional turmoil.

No one would argue that psychological factors per se determine whether you develop a herpes infection on your lip or genitals: this is a straightforward matter of exposure—the infection appears and generally recurs at the point where it entered the body. The two types of herpes affect people so differently because they tap into the very different meanings attached to the mouth and the genitals. Much suffering that accompanies genital herpes arises from the interaction between the disease itself and feelings of anxiety, guilt, and confusion about loving that we symbolically attach to the genital area.

Understanding "why there?" won't cure genital herpes. But understanding the complex emotions related to "there" may help you explore the emotional tasks that the herpes virus may be performing with frequent recurrences. This awareness has helped some patients end their recurrences.

Distinctions like "before the fact" and "after the fact" aren't always clear or important. But answering "why there?" will sometimes provide the essential clue to the symptom's psychological underpinning, or just add useful information to the clues you've been amassing with earlier exercises. If your skin problem has concentrated on one or several parts of your body, it's a question that no doubt has already occurred to you and is well worth asking.

Answering "why there?" means asking yourself what the afflicted body part means—to *you*. We use our bodies in common ways, so we share associations that give body parts a common meaning. Everyone talks, kisses, and eats with the mouth, so a rash here may suggest emotional conflicts involving communication or affection, for example.

But because our lives are different, we also develop our own set of personal, private associations: a rash on my arm may not mean to me what a rash on your arm means to you. The unique details of your life will give your body its unique symbolism. To a person who was often slapped across the mouth by an angry parent, a rash on the mouth will have a special meaning.

Answering "why there?" doesn't mean translating body parts into emotions using some kind of code book. It means thinking freely about your own experiences with, feelings about, and associations with the afflicted parts of your body. It means considering how you use your body in concrete, practical terms, as well as what your body means to you—what connotations and associations arise when you think of your hands, genitals, or whatever areas carry your symptom. It means thinking of your body in the context of your life and problems.

Mary G., for example, had a shy, lonely childhood. She had more than enough to cry about, but her stern, moralistic parents disparaged tears as a show of weakness. Now Mary was working with severely retarded, emotionally disturbed children—kids with profound problems of their own.

She came to me when her dermatologist could do little for a persistent rash that developed around her eyes. In therapy, it became clear that Mary empathically shared the sadness of the children she worked with; in their struggles she saw the pain of her own early years. It was enough to drive anyone to tears—but Mary's own tears were still dammed by her parents' injunctions. So the sadness expressed itself symbolically, in a rash that took the place of tears. As we explored the suppressed crying beneath the rash, Mary became able to confront her sad feelings directly. As she learned to cry real tears, her rash disappeared.

I want to stress again the personal nature of such body symbols; in another person, a similar rash might have a totally different meaning. The literature of psychopathology records the case of one woman who inadvertently witnessed her mother's infidelity. She developed a rash around the eyes that nearly closed them—an expression, perhaps, of the guilty feeling that she'd "seen too much," similar to the hysterical blindness we discussed earlier.

To appreciate the spectrum of meanings that attach to a single body part, let's consider several people who had trouble with their hands. We use our hands constantly, and a skin symptom there may reflect on any of these uses. We express anger with our hands; we fondle and masturbate; if we are "light-fingered" we steal with our hands. Metaphorically, we "handle" our lives, jobs, and relationships the way we handle objects, carefully, gracefully, tentatively, or awkwardly. If we have more than we can handle, we "have our hands full." If our needs are left unfilled, we come away "empty-handed."

Elsa D., a woman in her early twenties from a closely knit European family, aspired to be a concert violinist. But duty, according to her family's old-world values, demanded that she stay home to care for her elderly grandmother. She left for the conservatory anyway. But within a semester she was back home, forced to give up her studies by severe eczema on her hands.

Elsa's hands were caught in the squeeze between duty and personal aspiration: she felt guilty if she sought fulfillment on her own terms, angry at being trapped if she didn't. She could not allow herself to experience these "unacceptable" feelings.

The conflict between her own and her parents' values was all the more unresolvable because of Elsa's own conflicts about growing up and becoming independent. Her hands—which *would* play the violin, but *should* tend grandmother—became the battlefield of contradictory needs and demands.

Tom J. was a super-executive—a trouble-shooting expert hired by ailing companies to solve problems and bail them out. This time, however, it was clear he'd taken on a sinking ship: nothing he tried would pull off his customary miracle. Tom's trouble was compounded by turmoil at home: a stepson who was going through a particularly troubled adolescence.

The rash that developed on Tom's hands was mysterious.

Dermatological testing suggested he'd suddenly become allergic to common inks and papers. But even when he avoided them, the rash remained—even worsened. His hands, it seemed to me, were expressing a deeper problem: Tom's frustrated feeling that he'd failed to *handle* difficult situations in both his professional and personal life. Rather than take this blow to the ego directly, this man who was supposed to be able to "handle anything" took the rap symbolically.

Janet N. had been in psychotherapy for several years, when she developed a strange eczema that afflicted only the first finger of her right hand and the third finger of her left hand. As often happens in therapy, this woman had transferred to me strong emotions originally directed toward others. She wanted to be part of my real life, close to me in a way she'd never been allowed to be with her father. It seemed to me that the rash on her wedding finger and trigger finger pointed to the emotional hotbeds that had been aroused—her wish for closeness, along with anger at its frustration. Part of her wanted to marry me; another part to shoot me.

All three were quite successful in clearing their skins, once they discovered the metaphor.

Like these patients, you will only find the answer to "why there?" in your own experiences and problems. But the human condition that we share gives certain body areas a common ground of meaning, as widely understood figures of speech attest. This list of body associations is intended to stimulate, not replace, your own introspection. Think of it as an emotional map that suggests some places to look and some things to look for.

The *face* is the most visible organ. It is here our emotions are most flamboyantly displayed, voluntarily or despite our efforts to conceal them. Humiliated, we "lose face." Salvaging our pride, we try to "save face." The original stigma of guilt, the mark of Cain, appeared on the forehead.

The *mouth* is at the center of much emotion-laden experience—speaking, eating, kissing. It is a sensitive, expressive organ, deeply involved in sexuality. But the mouth is also an instrument of deception: the "lip service" we pay to ideas and feelings we don't truly believe in, the false smiles and frowns with which we deceive.

As an orifice, an opening, your mouth is a border station between you and the world. You take food in through your mouth, you breathe in and out. Consequently, it often has a symbolic role in emotional conflicts surrounding interactions with others, particularly when giving and getting are involved. This includes times when we "get" more than we want, when we're being unduly influenced and having things "rammed down our throats." Other orifices—ears, eyes, genitals, rectum—are also frequent symptom targets when these issues are involved.

The *eyes* are the source of tears and the organs with which we see—sometimes what we'd rather not. "Sight" is a frequent metaphor for perception and insight: we "lose sight of things" when we forget what's important and what's not. If we're greedy, overambitious, wanting more than we feel we have a right to, we have "big eyes." Gazing fixedly or deeply, we drink in the world with our eyes.

The *head* is where we think, and is thus a symbol of both intellection and disordered thought, brains and craziness. Overly intellectual types are said to live "from the neck up." Stubborn people are "headstrong" or "pigheaded"; the reckless go "head first"; to be overly proud is to have a "swelled head." Skin problems that focus on the head may suggest difficulties with self-esteem, with accepting intellectuality or keeping it from taking over.

The *hair* is the part of the body most easily lost, and feelings about loss are frequently expressed here. The biblical tale of Samson illustrates how hair can be a metaphor for potency. The whitening of hair is associated with wisdom, but also with aging, decline, and severe shock. The quick loss of hair can follow severe emotional stress.

The *chest* is the home of the heart, and when one's heart is breaking, the skin above it may actually break out. We associate the chest with the essential self, so getting something off it is a metaphor for confession, the expression of guilt. Sticking one's chest out is a confident assertion of self.

The *breasts* have sexual connotations as well as strong associations with nurturing and mothering. Our cultural obsession with breasts makes them symbols of attractiveness. Their usual concealment charges their display with emotion.

The *stomach* is below the chest, softer and more vulnerable—

a "soft white underbelly." It, like the chest, may be the meta-phorical heart of the person. Many cultures call the pit of the stomach the home of the soul; to the Japanese, it is the center of the vital life force *ki*. When we can't *stomach* something, literally or figuratively, the revulsion may be expressed on the skin of the stomach. The navel may symbolically maintain a lifelong link to mother.

Strong emotions, strong conflicts, and strong confusions are associated with the *genitals*. Unresolved feelings about loving and being loved may express themselves in genital skin problems. The genitals symbolize sexuality itself, and its echoes in assertiveness, attractiveness, and creativity. They may suffer when we have trouble exercising power. Many of us still have feelings of guilt associated with the genitals: this remains, in a corner of our minds, a taboo area.

Skin troubles around the *anus* or *buttocks* can express diffi-culty dealing with irritation—(witness the expression "pain in the ass"). Childhood feelings about dirtiness that we develop at the time of toilet training still cling to this area, in our minds, along with the emotionally tinged issue of self-control. Problems here may relate to sexual identity conflicts—homosexual fears or im-pulses we find too distressing to acknowledge. (One patient had recurrent warts in and around his anus, which served to sym-bolically protect him against the homosexual assault one part of him wished for, but another part feared with revulsion.)

Symptoms at the anus or farther up on the *back* may suggest conflicts about activity and passivity. Should we "back out" of our responsibilities? Bear burdens gladly? Go after what we want or just "sit on our ass"? A person hung up between active and passive, who resents his habitual passive role but cannot break out of it, may experience symptoms on his back.

We kick aggressively with our *legs* and *feet*. They are also the organs of locomotion and standing firm: they root us to the ground and give us the means to travel on—and may break out in a rash when we're unable to do either with ease. For one of my pa-tients, movement was a key feature of life. She never really planted herself firmly anywhere, but would move restlessly from one project, one relationship to another. Painful warts on her feet made it literally impossible for her to stand still and firm—and focused attention on this unresolved issue.

Putting one's foot down is an image of decisiveness, and foot problems may accompany difficulties in making decisions. The fact that they're "lower organs," pointy, moist, and sometimes odorous, can make them a symbol for the genitals, expressing conflicts and difficulties surrounding sex.

In asking your own "why there?" no guide can be better than your own associations, imagination, intuition. What does this part of your body, spotlighted by troubled skin, stand for? How does illness *there* feel different from illness elsewhere? All the great storehouses of metaphor and symbol—art, dreams, the language we use daily—may offer clues to the "thereness" that has become part of your troubled skin.

8

What Your Symptom Does for You

A paradox is something that seems absurd, impossible, or contradictory, but is actually true. When an intelligent person does something blatantly stupid, like running off with a man or woman everyone knows is shallow and devious and none too bright, that's a paradox. "The heart has its reasons," the French philosopher Pascal said centuries ago, "of which the reason knows nothing." A paradox can reveal an important truth that's hidden by logic.

If you have a chronic skin disease, you may be living with a paradox. You've probably gone to doctor after doctor to rid yourself of this affliction, which has disrupted your life and plans; you've tried vitamins, creams, lotions, and prayers. Now I'm asking you to believe that on one level you may *want* this problem, that there's a hidden part of yourself that *gains* from troubled skin. In addition to doing terrible things *to* you, I'm saying, your skin is doing things *for* you.

The self-knowledge exercises and the Animal Test of earlier chapters were designed to help put you in touch with an inner self you don't know at all well, whose emotional needs are somehow indirectly satisfied by your skin's illness—a part of you that *tells* your skin to be sick. Here we'll approach the mystery from the other side: what, more precisely, is your skin doing for that inner self?

First, let's confront this issue straight on, with a simple, straightforward exercise: *List ten advantages to your problem.*

Let's face it: if you take a broad enough view, virtually anything—any quandary, setback or disaster—holds an advantage of some sort. If you're going to be shot at dawn tomorrow, you won't have to worry about what to wear for lunch! The fundamental point of this exercise, like many in this book, is to shake up the black-and-white "good" and "bad" categories in which we usually pigeonhole life experiences. You're already all too aware of the enormous cost of your skin problem, in pain and disruption. To better understand its hold on you, let's explore the hidden profit in being sick.

If you get nothing out of this exercise but the breakthrough realization that your skin condition actually has advantages, you've accomplished a lot. You've started seeing it not merely as a curse to *get rid of*, but something that may linger until you're *ready to give it up*, like smoking or self-destructive relationships. Like many of my patients, you may find that you can't let go of your illness until you understand why you're holding on.

Most of us resist the notion that we're in any way *responsible* for our health problems. The line between responsibility and blame is easily blurred, and other people are all too ready to jump in and say "You really *want* to be sick" or "All you want is sympathy." Most understandably, anyone who has suffered for months or years with an intractable itch or rash wants her ordeal taken seriously and appreciated by friends and family. To suggest she has a stake in her illness, that there's gain along with pain, may threaten her sense of integrity.

It's nothing as simple or odd as wanting to be sick, of course, nor is a person who unwittingly abets the persistence of her illness "disturbed" or abnormal. Rather, her symptoms may be kept alive by part of her that wants what we all want—sympathy, comfort, and the rest—but unconsciously has chosen an unfortunate way to get it and keep it. In no sense is it a conscious strategy.

Here, we can learn much from recent pain research. Only in the last few years have doctors come to appreciate the mystery of what's called *chronic pain syndrome.* What happens here is that the pain of an injury endures long after the injury has healed.

Doctors can find no physical reason for the continuing pain, and they can do nothing to make it go away. Not long ago, sufferers from chronic pain were dismissed as hysterics and malingerers. Today, doctors recognize that they suffer as much as the victim of a migraine or slipped disk, and their pain is every bit as real.

While no one fully understands the cause of chronic pain, it seems that in some cases, at least, sufferers may in part be victims of a process that *trained* them to hold on to the pain.

Usually, the victim of an accident or injury is treated sympathetically and cared for. He often receives pain pills with pleasant side effects. If the legal system is involved, he may continue to receive money—but only as long as he suffers pain! In a very real sense, he is *rewarded* for having pain. On a fundamental level, the human organism and its muscles and nerves follow the same simple laws that rats, pigeons, and puppies follow—they keep on doing what they're rewarded for doing.[1]

Chronic pain victims don't say "I like this treatment, so I'm going to keep on feeling pain." They don't *want* to suffer any more than the rest of us. But—according to the theory, at least—they have been trained with psychological, even monetary, rewards to continue feeling pain. The "advantages" keep it hanging on.

There are many differences between pain and a rash or herpes outbreak; the point of the analogy is the *process*, the principle by which your body keeps on doing what it gets rewarded for, absurd and counterproductive as it may seem to your logical intelligence.

Often, psychologists and physicians made a useful distinction between *primary gain* and *secondary gain*. Primary gain is the heavy emotional push that gets psychosomatic symptoms started—the need to express anger that may eventuate in a rash, for example. Once the symptom has become interwoven into the fabric of life, it will probably bring along with it small but very real "fringe benefits": your illness will garner sympathy, and it may enable you to take more time off from work. These extra payoffs are *secondary gains*. You didn't ask for them, any more than you asked for your allergies or warts. They are the "bright side" of a very dark cloud. But the trouble is, they reward you for staying sick,

"My dermatologist is very nice and I get to see her regularly." For someone with an established skin problem, an ongoing relationship with a dermatologist can help keep it firmly entrenched. I've had socially isolated patients who freely admit that a regular visit to their dermatologist is the center of their social week. Many dermatologists and dermatological nurses are, in fact, very nice people, and certain therapeutic procedures, such as ultraviolet irradiation, can be quite pleasant. Most of us find it hard to take time out just to do something nice for ourselves, without a justification like illness. If you lose your skin condition, you may lose both a pleasant relationship with a caring doctor and time for self-pampering.

On the other hand, some skin patients get themselves into a kind of power struggle with the dermatologist (and some highly competitive or moralistic doctors seem to encourage this). You may be struggling to keep your symptom, much as when you were a child you struggled to express your natural independence against controlling, restrictive parents. Here, your skin becomes a costly battleground, where regular jousts provide a perverse satisfaction in defeating the doctor's best efforts.

"My severe dry skin means I can't wash the dishes." Concrete activity restrictions may be the most obvious kind of secondary gain. With a skin problem, as with any chronic illness, you're probably exempt from many boring, irritating chores—like the fellow with a dust allergy who was forbidden to vacuum by his allergist, and asked for a note to give his wife. No one would suggest that these very minor benefits outweigh the pain and suffering. They're little compensations, but they do reward you for remaining ill.

"I get to stay home from school." For many of us, social isolation represents a refuge from anxiety and conflict. If deeply seated in such emotional tasks as freezing time or avoiding sexual conflict, social isolation is a primary gain of skin illness. As a less intense but comforting way out of interpersonal demands, the ability to remain isolated can be a little reward of remaining ill—a secondary gain. It's also a satisfying way to retain control over one's life: a license to remain isolated *when we want to.*

"I couldn't possibly ask that girl out looking like this." An advan-

tage? The patient who listed this one added, "I'd love to ask her out . . . but I'm not sure I'd have the guts, even if I didn't look like this." Isolation and protection are the themes here, too; I've included it to point out that the hidden *profit* often looks very much like the *cost* of the illness. We want to do many things, but fear to try, or we feel wary about the results. Dating, for example, makes many people feel highly vulnerable—it arouses fear of rejection and challenges self-esteem, at the same time that it exerts its powerful attraction. If you've ever been paralyzed in ambivalence for long ("I want to . . . no, I don't . . . yes, I do . . .") you'll recognize this acute discomfort and the relief that comes when something beyond your control makes your mind up for you. A broken-out face removed this patient's uncertainty ("I can't . . ."), providing protection against risk along with a rationalization ("I would, if only my skin would clear up"). It's very common to ascribe to a skin problem our inability to do things we really don't want to do or fear doing. The next chapter's exercise is devoted, in part, to unmasking such self-deception.

"People are nice to me . . . I get lots of sympathy." For some, skin problems remain a permanent conversation piece, a constant stimulus to solicitous questions about their health and well-being. Instead of talking about the weather or baseball, they can talk about their skin, an advantage not to be dismissed lightly for those who have extreme difficulty making small talk and socializing.

Skin illnesses unquestionably garner sympathy. And sympathy is something we all need, in a world full of burdens and setbacks. Something as visible as problem skin will generate sympathy where less tangible troubles will not. There's nothing wrong with needing sympathy, of course—the problem is that this is a particularly costly way to get it.

"If I wasn't worrying about my skin, I'd probably be worrying about something even worse." This intriguing advantage came from a patient with unusual insight. We all have our share of free-floating dreads and anxieties, simply as part of our share in the human condition. A specific, concrete focus for our worries can, paradoxically, be helpful, even comforting. It *contains* our anxieties. While you're lying in bed trying not to scratch yourself into a bloody pulp, you won't be worrying about the unnamable things

that may be lurking in the dark around and within you.

"It provides something to focus my anger and disappointment on— something to bitch about." This actually contains two distinct advantages that many people find hard to separate in their minds.

Life is full of irritation and frustration, and most of us have a reservoir of anger that sometimes demands release. Often we displace our anger on those close to us—the classic example being the man or woman who comes home from a frustrating day at the office and starts yelling at the kids. A chronic skin condition is a safe, guilt-free, and reliable target for the discharge of anger.

Disappointment is more complex. Many people fasten on one turning point in their lives where it all went wrong—where they went off the track and slipped irretrievably toward failure. The classic example is the former boxer played by Marlon Brando in the movie *On the Waterfront*. Some time before the movie takes place, Brando threw a fight, his career went off the rails, and his whole life, in his mind, went into a nose dive that he could never pull up out of. "I coulda been a contender, instead of a bum, which is what I am," he mutters. A patient of mine, a lawyer, felt the same way about the fact that he couldn't get into the Ivy League college he preferred, and had to settle for a (to him) third-rate institution. Thus he was condemned to lifelong mediocrity, out of the mainstream.

It's illogical, of course, but there's satisfaction in the ability to focus one's disappointment in life on a single event or situation and say, "There. That's where I lost it, and that's that." Counting oneself out of life, you can stop struggling, and for many people the single accepted blow is easier to bear than life's repeated affronts to ambition and sense of self. The development of a serious skin problem can become, in the mind, just such a turning point, "and that's that."

"It hurts so nice when I scratch." This surprising response points out that there is a very real satisfaction—almost a sexual one—in the immediate relief you get from scratching an itch. In fact, "scratching where it itches" is a figure of speech for satisfaction. (Squeezing pimples and tearing off scabs provide similar pleasure—although many adults find it hard to admit.) The moments of intense relief don't balance the tormented hours of itching, but

they do give periodic gratifications that one can look forward to.

"The boss knows I'll be out from time to time. Otherwise, he'd give me grief if I asked for days off." Not only do people give you sympathy when you're ill, they give you special consideration. We can all use occasional "mental health days" when we aren't expected to show up for work. Unfortunately, all we're entitled to are "sick days." A chronic illness means allowances are made for your special needs—a privilege that is understandably hard to give up.

"It gives me an excuse to avoid lovemaking with my husband." It's been said that "I have a headache" is quickly being replaced by "My herpes is active" as a sexual sidestep. Here again we're dealing with an advantage that's often well hidden. We like to think of ourselves as highly sexed beings—many men in particular have been led to expect themselves to perform like a furnace with a pilot light that's always burning. For a whole host of reasons, ranging from deep-seated sexual conflicts to fatigue, worry, and the vagaries of daily life, we may not be as eager for sex as our self-image demands.

The pain, irritation, or annoyance of an established skin condition provides a convenient rationale for avoiding sex without raising self-doubts about one's sexuality or getting into lengthy discussions on the nuances of your relationship.

"I have a whole wardrobe of special fabrics, which would be wasted if I didn't have an allergy." This is to remind you to include the seemingly trivial with the serious, in considering those advantages that keep you holding on to your skin troubles. The lightest additional weight swings the balance toward illness and away from health. In compiling your list, include even the most easily overlooked fringe benefits you give if your skin troubles continue, and try to imagine the most minor, inconsequential difficulty that will ensue if it improved.

Because they're important so often, I'd like to mention two other areas in which secondary gains can keep skin problems holding on: love and money.

People typically lapse into customary roles in long-standing relationships, particularly marriage: one person is the leader, the other the follower; one is the dreamer and the other the voice of reality. In some marriages, one partner takes the sick role, the other is the healthy spouse, and this becomes a fundamental basis of the relationship. It's a medium of giving and receiving affection, a division of power, a constant shared interest and a way to avoid conflict. If the sick spouse suddenly threw away his crutches (or her steroid creams) and became whole, the whole marriage would have to be reshuffled and redefined—a frightening prospect.

Money can also complicate skin problems. A full half of workers' compensation claims involve skin conditions. There's nothing phony or trumped-up about such claims, and few if any claimants are sick for profit. Rather, the high rate of skin problems authentically related to working conditions and office and industrial chemicals testifies to the callous disregard of workers' health that has long characterized American business.

Anyone whose health has been tarnished by his work fully deserves compensation. But it carries a hidden tax. No matter how the condition started, no matter how eager and willing you'd be to exchange a compensation check for your original health, as long as you receive money for being ill, this "reward" can be a powerful weight in the balance to keep you from getting well.

In doing the "advantages" exercise, a key is to suspend your normal commonsense notions about proportion and cause-and-effect. You're not *consciously* staying sick to reap these rewards: logic isn't what's holding them on, so logic can't always figure them out. These are simply the small, unasked-for dividends you get on a very large expense of energy and pain. Even the smallest of them add to the forces that keep your skin troubled, opposing the difficult work of change to make it better. And while they may be easier to unearth than the emotional tasks in which your skin problem may be more deeply rooted, they can persist with a tenacity completely out of proportion to their real-life importance.

Don't be troubled or blocked by the sense that these advantages are base or unworthy. Again, they correspond to needs we all have—for love, for protection, for respect—and you're certainly getting them the hard way. Even advantages that seem dubious to you, like attracting attention or receiving sympathy, should be considered seriously. There may be a part of you that revels in sympathy, even while your stoic self recoils. Above all, remember the differences between taking responsibility and blaming yourself.

As with the deeper emotional tasks, bringing these advantages to light is a first step. If you learn to gain similar satisfactions straightforwardly, you'll weaken the hold of your illness—you won't "need" to be sick. For example, if you recognize that your relationship with your dermatologist or her periodic treatments are a significant reward for your illness, consider alternatives: other relationships that may fill the same need, such as an ongoing involvement with the dermatology clinic as a volunteer.

If you've had a serious skin problem for some time, you may be surprised to discover how your skin has become a tyrant, dictating much of your life. The problem is *there*, and so it's taken on the satisfaction of various needs that you might well resolve in healthier ways if it were not. How would you live without it? One step toward making the secondary gains of illness unnecessary is to *imagine* what life would be like if your skin cleared entirely. In particular, this will help clear away the self-deceptions that give certain of the gains we've discussed their power. This, in fact, is the subject of the next exercise.

9

What If It Got Better?
A Good News–Bad News
Story

Suppose your prayers were answered. When the clock struck midnight you felt a tingle all over and . . . Shazam! your skin problems were gone. All gone! Your skin was fine and healthy from head to toe. Wouldn't that be wonderful? All your troubles would be over!

Don't be so sure. Look at all your friends with healthy skin: are they perfectly happy? Was your life a bowl of cherries before your skin started giving you grief? The point of this exercise is realism—not to rain on your parade, but to help you appreciate what role your skin symptom plays in your life, and what role it *doesn't* play. The question "What if it got all better?" is another way to get a handle on *what your problem is doing for you,* and to help you know it well enough to let it go.

Sit down and ask yourself: "What if my skin disease were suddenly cured at midnight?"—or noon, if you prefer daytime miracles. "How would my life be different?" Make a solid effort to imagine your life without troubled skin. You'd still get up in the morning and brush your teeth, but perhaps you'd spend less time looking ruefully in the mirror. You'd still eat breakfast. You'd still dress (but would you wear the same clothes?). Go through your daily routine in fantasy, noting how it would change in big and little ways. Take notes.

Freely imagine all the areas of your life that would change.

What would you do *then* that you can't do *now?* What would happen to your relationships with other people? To your work? Your friendships? Your sex life?

The first payoff of this exercise is simple. It's hard to accomplish what you can't imagine, and forming a clear mental picture (it will probably grow clearer as you practice the exercise over time) is an important first step to making a dream come true: this is the true power of "positive thinking." Physiologically, our bodies respond to imaginary life much as they respond to real life, and imagination is in a great rehearsal stage. In doing this exercise, you are *rehearsing* healthy skin.

But the exercise can do more. Looking closely at the dreams-come-true that follow your imaginary total recovery, you'll tap into the fantasy world of emotions that got your symptom started, heightens it, and keeps it hanging on.

Thirty-five-year-old Andrew M. came in for psychotherapy for a different problem, but it was immediately evident that his acne caused him great distress. He had had a severe case on his face and his back since his early teens. While exploring his feelings about this symptom, I raised the question: "What if it suddenly got better?"

For one thing, Andrew said, he could leave his girlfriend, with whom he'd been living for two years. This desire to part hadn't come up in our earlier sessions; as we explored it further, it came out that while Andrew was quite fond of Jane, she was—well, plain. She was attractive enough, bright, caring, creative—but she just wasn't the girl of his dreams, the glamorous, sexy woman he imagined as his proper partner . . . the girl he could get *if only* his skin were not such a mess!

If only! We'll return to this magic phrase shortly, and dwell on it at length. For now, let's consider the truth about Andrew and Jane. There was a sense, he admitted, in which he was angry at his hapless housemate for being just herself—for not having the larger-than-life sparkle he craved; for not being, as he put it, "a prom queen."

Dating the luminous prom queen, the movie star, was, I pointed out, a delightful and nearly universal fantasy, but at root an adolescent one. There was something adolescent, too, in some of Andrew's other fantasies of what he'd do *if only* his skin cleared. He could travel widely. He could run for public office. He could do just about anything. If only his skin would let him.

In fact, the fantasy world that Andrew brought forth was more or less the dream of unlimited potential that properly belongs to the high school years. The adolescent is full of potential: he's not yet fully formed and he hasn't chosen his path through life. In theory, he can be an astronaut or president. Andrew had a particularly strong reason to freeze time and remain an adolescent in spirit: his true adolescence had been stunted and blighted by serious family turmoil and divorce. He'd spent his high school days sad and isolated.

Although the acne had troubled him for years, Andrew had given up on dermatologists—and this in itself suggested that something in him wanted, needed, to hold on to the problem. His disease, acne, symbolically extended adolescence. Equally important, it cushioned reality to protect his treasured sense of adolescent potentiality. No, perhaps he wasn't living with a movie star; and his job, while respectable, was neither exciting nor glamorous. Sure, he was living an ordinary life like millions of other ordinary folks, equally ignored by *People* magazine and *Who's Who*. But this was only because his skin prevented him from realizing his true potential.

Andrew's acne was explicitly bound up with the emotional task of freezing time and maintaining adolescence, but this particular role, the buffer between the real world and precarious self-esteem, is shared by many dissimilar skin problems. Bad skin can be a permanent exemption from the testing process that life constantly inflicts on our self-image.

If only the lupus went away, we'd look good enough to attract rich, caring men. *If only* that maddening itch would quit, we could devote our energies to our studies and graduate *summa cum laude*. *If only* the warts shriveled up, we could be happy! We all achieve some dreams and have to forget others, and life being what it is, we inevitably fall short of the satisfaction we crave. But when self-esteem is fragile, such setbacks are too heavy to handle. Instead, we tell ourselves: "I could do it, I could have done it, I *would* do it—if only my skin would let me!"

Bad skin is only one resource we use to shore up our egos.

We fall prey to similar self-deceptions when we tell ourselves: "If only I could get it together and move to California—then life would be great," or "If only I had ten thousand dollars—then I could take a year off and write the novel I know I could write if I didn't have to earn a living," or "If only I could find the right man/woman (or if the man/woman I've got now would disappear) I could be happy and fulfilled." They are all one-shot simplistic explanations to excuse why we haven't become the person we want to be or that someone said we should be. They mask the complex push-and-pull, the needs and fears that make "what we want to be" so complicated and that make its achievement so difficult. The skin is a particularly convenient and convincing "if only." It can serve this purpose indefinitely.

A major goal of this exercise is to bring the "if only" ways you rely on your troubled skin out into the open, to help you judge for yourself how much of your healthy-skin fantasies have a basis in reality. Look closely and honestly at your fantasies of a new life. Are they realistic? To what extent are you *fooling yourself* that life would be radically improved? Remember: self-deception isn't an innocent past time. Your ability to preserve illusions about "the real you" is one of the advantages that may keep your skin problem hanging on.

If you do this exercise with sensitivity and imagination, you can dig deeper than self-image protection. "If only" fantasies express wishes; these, as we've discussed earlier, are sisters under the skin to fears. And understanding both can illuminate the hotbeds of emotional action that stir up symptoms and keep them active.

When I asked one of my patients what he could do if his dermatitis cleared, he answered: "If I didn't have that constant, draining aggravation, I could get it together and start my own business!" As he said it—and imagined the process—he noted within himself a wave of anxiety along with the pleasant feelings of pride and achievement. As you imagine life without your skin affliction, be sensitive to your own feelings: the same shiver of fear may pass over you as you imagine, "I could date lovely women," or "I could set out with a backpack and hike the Appalachian Trail, alone."

Your problem skin may be the most visible obstacle between

you and your ambitions, but behind that are very likely subtler, deeper impediments—fears and anxieties. By stripping away the obvious obstacle, in imagination, this exercise brings you face to face with them. Anxiety is such an uncomfortable state that we'll go to great lengths to avoid it. Remember the fellow in last chapter's exercise who listed "I can't ask that beautiful woman out with my face like this" as an advantage of his eczema? He understood that his skin was protecting him against his anxieties. It's a secondary gain of many skin disorders.

Once more we're in the closed circle of paradox, where wishes and fears, drawbacks and advantages come together. The thing you *would* do with healthy skin—go after sex, success, or adventure, for example—is something you're *not doing* today. Why not? Is there something under your skin stopping you, a fear masked by the obvious obstacle? Is your skin, perhaps, actually resolving the conflict between the part of you that wants to go after sex, success, or adventure and the part that is afraid to try? For example, if you fantasized that with healthy skin, you could "go out and have a busy, satisfying social life," you should at least consider the paradoxical possibility that your skin isn't *inflicting* isolation on you, but *allowing* you to isolate yourself and avoid the anxieties of social contact.

There's a human tendency to lump separate problems together, a process I call *agglomeration*. A person who is troubled by severe acne and who has fewer friends than she wants will say: "I don't have any friends because my skin looks so terrible." Only after a period of soul searching may it become clear that she had as few friends *before* her skin troubles started. This is something to ask yourself as you go through the "what if it got better" exercise. Did you do the things you yearn for (date handsome men/lovely women, start your own business, travel the world) *before* you developed your problem? Are they really out of the question with your skin as it is now? Are your unsatisfied ambitions and problem skin, in fact, two different things?

You must untangle the agglomeration of skin problems and other problems if you want to work on either effectively. Lumped together, allergic dermatitis, feelings of isolation, and a fear of sexual encounters form a mountain of difficulty so massive that any attempt to scale it is doomed. Only by separating them can you cut it down to size. It's like any big project: wake up and think of cleaning your entire apartment, and your instinct may well be to curl up under the covers indefinitely. But break it up into manageable steps—pile up the newspapers, take them out, vacuum the living room, dust the furniture—and it begins to seem not easy, perhaps, but possible.

With Dan G., a twenty-two-year-old contractor from western Massachusetts, separating a big problem into its component parts was a dramatic therapy breakthrough. Dan, a quiet, socially isolated fellow who lived with his parents, had painful, persistent warts on his hands. They interfered with his work, and his dermatologist was powerless to help. In sheer numbers they were overwhelming—layers and layers of warts that made their treatment wart by wart unthinkable.

At first, therapy went smoothly. A single session in which we used hypnosis relieved the pain of the warts. But the warts themselves hung in there. They remained through months of psychotherapy, through repeated hypnotic sessions where I used every unblocking technique I knew.

After a frustrating year, I was trying to help Dan get in touch with his feelings with a technique called the Inner Adviser, which aims to set up a dialogue with the deepest parts of the self (you'll learn about this in detail in a later chapter). Under hypnosis, I asked why progress was so slow. What would happen, I asked, if the warts went away? The answer was finally released: "I'd have to deal with the problem of going out with women."

It had long been clear that dating made Dan apprehensive, and that his sexual experiences had been generally disappointing. He'd had few girlfriends. But it was difficult for him to *admit* that he was lonely, that he wanted to go out more—this would amount to admitting he was a failure, rather than a bit of a loner who could take women or leave them alone. Having a satisfying social and sexual life had never been made an "official" goal.

What snapped into place now was the extent to which the warts and the social problem had become connected in Dan's mind. If the warts went away, he'd have to face the demands of dating— or explaining to himself why he didn't date—head on. Taken together, warts and dating were a big mountain of a problem. The stakes were too big, and it felt as if his only option was to hold on to the warts.

Once the connection was out in the open, I suggested a deal to Dan. We agreed that his skin had nothing to do with dating. Warts were warts, and women were women: if the warts went away, it put Dan under no obligation to resolve his dating dilemmas. Progress on the warts wouldn't force the issue: he'd go out when he was ready.

The agreement was a true breakthrough. The warts disappeared within three visits (a quick response not atypical with this condition), and then we started—slowly and sensitively—to work on Dan's troubled feelings about himself and women.

For Dan, progress became possible when he could hear the question "What would happen if your warts went away?" and answer it, *"I just wouldn't have them anymore and that's all."* This is ultimately the point of this exercise and in a way the goal of this whole part of the book: to lead you toward a realization that your skin is properly one thing, and your underlying psychological difficulties something else; and that your mind, which yoked them together, can also take them apart. I want you to accept that if your eczema cleared by a midnight miracle, or your allergies diminished, or your herpes recurrences became mild and infrequent, your life would certainly be more pleasant. But this wouldn't solve your other problems. You'd still have to get on with the business of living: overcome your nervousness about starting your own business; work out the fears of rejection that make you reluctant to date.

As you learn to see what your mind has attached to your skin problem, the symptom itself will become lighter. Ironically, when there's less at stake in losing the problem, it's easier to lose—as it's easier to set down a half-pound bag of oranges than a fifty-pound bag of cement. Without the burden of all your needs and emotional tasks, your skin problem will become a shell of itself. When you can see that the statement "I can't go out looking like this" expresses two unrelated problems—"I can't go out" and "I look like this"—you can start working to resolve each in turn.

10

What If It Got Worse?

What if my skin got worse? You must have asked yourself this question before, in terror that you haven't yet seen the bottom of the barrel. "My God," it's natural to ask when yet another treatment fails, "what if it got worse?"

When you remove the desperation you have a serious, profitable line of inquiry, just as you did when you seriously asked yourself "Why me?" Imagining an answer to the question "What if it got worse?" is like putting your skin under a psychological microscope. Everything is enormously enlarged—the pain, but also the gain. To answer the question honestly means following your deepest fears all the way down to their dreadful nadir. It is on this emotional ground that you'll find the secret wishes at the bottom of your illness.

This exercise is hard because it's scary. There's a nearly universal fear that imagining something can make it happen. This is akin to the "magical thinking" responsible for superstitions, for childhood games like pretending that if you step on a crack you'll break your mother's back, and for emotional problems like compulsion and guilt. Why stir up trouble by thinking terrible thoughts?

Besides pointing out that you already have trouble (why else are you reading the book?), I want to reassure you. To the best of my knowledge, nobody has *ever* made a skin illness worse simply by doing this exercise. The emotions that hurt are the ones we refuse to imagine, not the images we confront bravely and openly. In fact, getting strongly emotional material out from under your skin is what this book is all about, and for many people, carrying through with this exercise is a significant victory. If you can break through your fear of the unknown, think the unthinkable, and see that lightning does *not* strike you down, you've struck a major blow for emotional freedom. What you actually discover about the pains and gains of your illness may be less significant than the self-mastery you practice in making yourself able to face the question squarely.

One fair warning about flare-ups. Many chronic skin conditions, like other chronic illnesses, vary from day to day, week to week: they flare up and then cool down. As you get seriously into this and the other self-diagnosis exercises, you may find that your skin problem does flare up. Don't be surprised and don't be scared. It's just another way in which your mind defends its secrets, the emotional material it does not want found. Such flare-ups are in fact encouraging: they suggest that you are on the right track. As you get closer to the problem, it warns you away and buries itself deeper.

These flare-ups are invariably short-lived and will just fade into the illness cycle of ups and downs. It's the long run that we're concerned about: if you yourself can make your skin worse, that's a clear sign that you can make it better.

The actual exercise is simplicity itself. All you do is ask the same question, over and over: "What if it got worse?" Let one image be the jumping-off spot for the next, as you imagine your skin's progressive deterioration, and its effect on your life. What makes it difficult is the pain associated with such fantasies—they aren't anything you enjoy thinking about. And because it's a good question—good at unearthing hidden needs and unfinished emotional tasks—it will generate resistance from within. Your inner self will agree, "Let's not think about it."

"What if it got worse?" This is not a riddle to ask and answer intellectually. You answer it by *living* it mentally, imagining your skin getting worse the same way you might daydream about a warm Caribbean beach in January. Being there in your head.

There's no strict 1-2-3 method: everyone has his or her own fantasy style. Have you ever imagined a showdown with a manipulative relative or exploitative boss, and felt your pulse race in anger? When some get seriously into the imaginative work of this exercise, they feel the same anxiety and distress that would accompany a real skin worsening—along with the subtler emotions they're trying to understand.

There are others who ask themselves the question fancifully, letting their minds toss out bizarre, fantastic images till one hits home. Many a truth is spoken in jest.

Some of my patients have found work on this exercise goes quickly: they're ready to make themselves better, and the emotional secrets of their symptom have come so close to the surface that they can be quickly exposed. But it's more often a lengthy process. "What if it got worse?" is a question you may have to live with for a time, asking it relentlessly, day by day. Get the perspectives of different times of day, different moods. When an image strikes you with the ring of truth, you may want to enter it in your notebook. But don't stop there: Keep on pushing for the next.

One of my patients, John P., had been tormented by intractable itching for years. It came and went, but stayed long enough for him to scratch his body raw. When I asked him, "What if it got worse?" he answered, "I'd itch *all* the time." Then: "It would spread over my entire body."

What would this mean? I asked. "I wouldn't be able to work."

So? What if it got even worse?

"My wife would have to do all the chores and spend all the rest of her time taking care of me." This, we agreed, was an interesting image. My patient's fear of disability had been clear all along, but now its other side emerged: the powerful *wish* to be loved and cared for—an emotional task left over from childhood.

But we didn't stop there. When I urged him to imagine his condition still worse, a wholly different theme emerged. After all the dermatologists in New York, Boston, and Chicago failed to cure him, "They'd have to call in the super-expert consultant of consultants."

What then? "I'd frustrate the hell out of the bastard. He'd get back into his private jet and fly home in absolute disgrace."

And if it got still worse? "I'd scratch myself into a bloody pulp, a real bundle of pain. Everyone who saw me would be overwhelmed with sympathy. They'd set up a charitable foundation to support and treat me!" What now became clear was the close tie between his need for love and nurturing and the deeply held belief that these can only be won through suffering.

The frustrated experts and authorities and the angry tone of voice in which John described them pointed to his deep rage at their failure to him. They were like parents who didn't come through. But there was something more. John P. clearly derived real satisfaction from frustrating the experts' efforts. Part of him was in competition with those he asked for help (perhaps because he resented the need for *anyone's* help) and had a stake in their failure. But the only way for him to win this competition was to keep on itching and suffering. With an understanding of the need for love that fueled his illness and the anger that undercut the help he sought, John could begin to satisfy his needs more directly.

With John P., the "What if it got worse?" process unfolded over a period of three weeks. When you work on this exercise on your own, you should allow at least that long. Twice daily, sit down and give it serious attention.

Where, when, and how is a matter of personal style. Where would you go to do creative work (writing a letter to a friend on a sensitive subject, for example)? Where would you *imagine* yourself writing a poem, painting a picture, composing a musical score? Do you feel most creative sitting in the park? In an upstairs room with four white walls and little furniture? Next to a window with a view? Some people make creative headway while driving to work or while running. Try different settings for different perspectives. Most people do best when comfortable and isolated from the demands and distractions of everyday life. You shouldn't have to worry about the phone while you're letting your thoughts and feelings drift.

What time is most creative for you? The imagination works best in the early morning, for some, while others are at their sharpest between dinner and bedtime. (The essential thing, though,

is to do it *sometime*. Anyone can come up with practical reasons why they can't: "I'd love to concentrate on the exercise in the early morning, but it's such a rush to get to work, and my evenings are always busy.")

One trick that may shake up your creative powers, for this or any exercise, is to force yourself out of your usual thinking habits. Do you sit on questions endlessly, mulling them over before trying to solve them? This time, drive yourself hard, pushing for direct answers with a minimum of contemplation. If you typically push for quick answers and snap decisions, slow down and mull things over.

This exercise is a mental dialogue—a therapy session is which one part of your mind is the "therapist" and the other is the "patient" or "client." You can make the dialogue more realistic by imagining a real person repeating "What if it got worse?" over and over. Summon up the image of a supportive but persistent person, perhaps a key figure in your life. Who do you think would be most able to get straight answers out of you?

The most effective way to do this exercise may be with the help of a real person, perhaps a trustworthy and sensitive friend or family member who will do the asking. There's significant value simply in sharing your self-help efforts with someone close, in expressing the thoughts and needs you've buried because they seemed forbidden, and seeing that you're not rejected or punished.

How will you feel as images of deepening illness unfold? The emotional level of your response is critical. "Listening" to what your inner self tells you is like listening to the radio: if the message is too soft, you can't hear it; but if it's too loud, you'll hear nothing but a buzz of noise. An unemotional reaction to the question "What if it got worse?" is a kind of resistance: many people intellectualize such questions, detaching their emotions from their fantasies for self-protection. But an emotional overload of anxiety or despair may be another defense—a smokescreen of feeling to hide the details and subtleties.

If your emotional level seems low-key when you're doing this exercise, try coming back to it when you're already upset about overdue bills, or when a hard day at the office has tightened your

nerves to a high pitch. On the other hand, if you find yourself so upset at the exercise that you can't think straight, come back when you're calmer. Look for times when you're particularly relaxed and mellow.

Progress comes gradually to most, but some experience dramatic breakthroughs. For months, one of my patients had struggled to clarify the feelings of vulnerability beneath the rash that had seriously impaired her ability to live a normal adult life. "What if it got worse?" I asked her—not for the first time.

"I'd be immobilized," she said. "I wouldn't even be able to walk. I wouldn't be able to talk!"

And worse? "I wouldn't even be able to eat by myself. I couldn't lift a fork."

Worse still?

"Even the air would be dangerous to me. Dust and air pollution could damage my raw skin."

Worse? "I'd have to be put in a special plastic sack, filled with warm, soothing cream. I'd have to be fed by a tube. No one could come near me, except for the one person who knew how to operate the sack. She would feed me through the tube. I could do nothing except lie there, suspended in the soothing cream. There would be no demands, no responsibilities—

"My God!" my patient said abruptly. "Do you know what that sounds like? Back to the womb. That's *one* time my mother came through for me. Am I trying to get back there? Does that make sense?"

Not to the reason, perhaps, but to the heart. An early lack of nurturing love left her with a lifelong hunger that could swallow up her whole life before it was filled. What would make sense to both heart and reason, I suggested, would be to begin the painful process of mourning the little girl who was never loved. This woman went on to confront the deep source of her sadness directly, and to start building a life in which some of her need for love would be satisifed in healthier ways.

PART TWO

What You
Can *Do*
About It

11

The Healing State: Your Untapped Resource

Do you ever get so absorbed in a piece of music or a knotty problem that you fail to notice when a friend enters the room? Have you ever felt your mind float as your muscles melted in a hot bath or sauna? Then you're already familiar with a mental medicine that can do for your skin what stress has done against it.

I've paid a lot of attention to the down side of the mind-skin link. First were the needs, fears, and conflict that act themselves out in skin language: the sexual anxiety underneath Don's recurrent herpes, the cry for love frozen in Carol's eczema. Then came stress, the wear and tear of everyday hassles plus the strenuous gear-shifting that accompanies all of life's losses and wins, from birth to death with a hundred varied changes in between.

You may wonder if you wouldn't be better off without a mind, or perhaps with a mind kept in a state of dulled-out tranquillity: that way there'd be no stress and emotion to keep your skin fired up. But life as a vegetable isn't the answer. You can only avoid stress entirely if you avoid *life* entirely—too high a price, even for skin as satiny as an eggplant's.

Not that you have a choice. To be human is to have feelings, needs, and fears—to suffer as well as dance and smile. There's nothing to gain by pretending they're not there. What you need is an antidote that will let you experience life fully yet spare your skin the physiological consequences of life's unavoidable stress. Here's good news and more good news: not only does such an antidote exist, you already have it within you. It's just a question of learning to *activate and liberate* your mind's natural abilities.

You've probably heard of "altered states of consciousness" perhaps in the context of drug trips and bizarre experiences. Actually, the phrase simply refers to those states of mind that are neither the normal attentiveness of waking life, nor sleeping, nor dreaming. They include highly positive states, such as the exaltation that comes when we lose ourselves in great music, and very painful experiences such as panic and acute grief. We slip in and out of altered states dozens, perhaps hundreds of times each day.[1]

Certain of these states not only feel good, but are good for you. They can bring relaxation, diversion from care, and heightened control over your body—including your skin. The most familiar of these "healing states" is daydreaming. As you let your mind drift while you gaze out the window, the usual distracting crossfire of thoughts, plans, memories, and worries is hushed: although daydreaming sounds like inattention, it is actually a state of highly focused attention—on a fantasy. In this state, your mind becomes more imaginative: you think more creatively than logically, more in images than words. Half an hour may pass unnoticed, or a lengthy fantasy may unroll in minutes.

We enter similar states while engrossed in reading, while running, biking, or walking, while driving or soaking in the tub. They're a kind of vacation from the normal cares of the day— and more. With a little training and effort, you can learn to harness this focused mind energy for health. Used properly, this healing state is a tool to relieve skin symptoms and to help you explore the emotional turmoil beneath them. In this chapter, you will learn how to tap into the healing state at will; in chapters to come, to go beyond this state to use techniques that will intensify benefits for your skin.

The most immediate benefit of healing-state exercises is relaxation. In his book *The Relaxation Response* Dr. Herbert Benson of Harvard Medical School has identified the physical response evoked by such activities: muscles loosen, breathing deepens, heartbeat slows, and blood pressure drops.[2] This relaxation response is the physiological opposite of stress, and so I advocate daily practice of a healing state exercise to neutralize the unavoidable stress of your life, and help prevent your emotions from kicking your skin around.

Dr. Benson points out that most traditional cultures have their own ways of inducing the relaxation response. Meditation and prayer may primarily be ways to pursue harmony with the universe or communion with God, but both also evoke this body-sparing reaction. It seems that all cultures recognize the need for a break from mundane reality, and have built it into daily routine, as sound traditional diets quietly satisfy the need for protein, vitamins, and minerals.

In our high-speed, high-tech world, relaxation breaks have gone the way of the well-balanced diet. Many of the things we do to relax—such as watching football on TV—are actually stress-producing, and chemical relaxation with tranquilizers or alcohol take their own toll. For this reason, many health-minded people conscientiously include daily relaxation exercises in their lives, the same way they make a special effort to get exercise and to eat nourishing foods.

There are a number of widely used, easily learned techniques to gain the benefits of relaxation. They include autogenics, Jacobson's progressive relaxation, meditation, and self-hypnosis. If you've had good experience with any of these, you can use them now. If not, here are two exercises I've found simple and serviceable.

THE BENSON TECHNIQUE

When Dr. Benson surveyed the various ways that different cultures brought on the relaxation response, he discovered a few essential elements they had in common. They involved a symbol to focus on, or a word, sound, or phrase to repeat. They were practiced on a comfortable but not sleep-inducing position (people who sit, kneel, or squat at prayer or meditation can't doze off), and in a quiet environment outside the flow of daily life.

Dr. Benson combined these elements into a nonsectarian relaxation procedure—a kind of meditation without spiritual content. It's quite simple:

1. Sit in a quiet place where you won't be disturbed by ringing phones or other interruptions. Close your eyes. Let all your muscles loosen and relax. Relax the muscles of your feet, then work up all through your body, a wave of relaxation gradually coming up to your face. Breathe evenly through your nose, and become aware of the intake and outflow of each breath.

2. As you breathe out, say the word "one" to yourself. Let a comfortable, regular rhythm establish itself: breathe in, breathe out, "one"; in, out, "one." Breathe easily and naturally.

3. A passive attitude is important. Don't worry about being successful, and don't monitor your state of relaxation. Let the relaxation response develop at its own pace. You're not really *doing* it—just observing what your body's doing. Distracting thoughts and fantasies will enter your head. Ignore them, without struggling to push them away. Keep on repeating "one" to yourself and they will drift out again.

Do the exercise for ten or fifteen minutes or as long as seems comfortable. You may want a watch or clock in a handy position so you can check the time just by opening your eyes. Don't use an alarm.

When you conclude the exercise, sit quietly for several minutes, first with your eyes closed, then with your eyes open, as you slowly return to ordinary consciousness and ordinary life. Take a few more minutes before you stand up and get back to your routine.

Dr. Benson recommends doing the exercise once or twice a day. He feels that digestion interferes with the response, and suggests waiting two hours after eating.

SELF-HYPNOSIS

This is an excellent way to gain the relaxation benefits of the healing state, and possibly the best preparation for the treatment exercises to come. It's the technique I've found most valuable in working with my patients.

Regrettably, hypnosis still retains a magic-show aura that keeps many from appreciating its possibilities. No, hypnosis does not mean a Svengali putting dupes under his power, making them cluck like chickens and perform ridiculous stunts they'd never do while "awake." In fact, it's not something that somebody does *to you* at all, but something you do *for yourself*, perhaps with the help of another person.

Hypnosis is a trance state—an altered state of consciousness related to the absorption in music and daydreams we flit into and out of throughout the day. The movie audience so focused on the screen that the rest of the world fades away is actually in a very similar trance. With hypnosis, however, concentration can be so focused that you are able to change physiology and perception. People who are able to enter a very deep trance can have surgery with no anesthesia besides hypnosis. For me this is like seeing airplanes fly and babies being born. I've seen it, I know the theory, but I don't quite believe it.

Scientists remain mystified by the versatility of hypnosis. It may produce profound relaxation (we're going to use it this way), but the trance itself is not always a relaxed state—you can be hypnotized while pedaling a bicycle. There are no body changes that always happen in hypnosis. You can tell whether a person is awake or asleep by looking at his brain waves on an electro-encephalogram, for example, but not whether or not he is hypnotized.

The ability to enter a hypnotic trance seems largely inborn: 25 percent of adults can go into deep trances, 25 percent are capable only of a very light trance (simply pleasant relaxation), and the rest of us fall somewhere in between. There's no clear connection between intelligence, sex, personality, and trance capacity, but it seems that people with vivid imaginations—the kind who had imaginary playmates in childhood—are likeliest to have good hypnotic ability. Our skill usually peaks at ages eight to ten.[3]

Motivation is an important factor. With a big stake in success, you can achieve a trance to the utmost of your capacity: a strong desire to improve your skin can be instrumental in gaining good results.

While the experience is dramatic for some, even people who

only slip into light trances often achieve major benefits. "Is that all there is?" certain patients have asked me, incredulous that what seems like a ho-hum experience can bring such help to their skin.

My patients are often surprised when I tell them that hypnosis is something they can do themselves, that it does not require the help of an anointed expert. Actually, the difference between hypnosis and self-hypnosis is just the difference between entering the same trance state with help and doing it on your own. There are any number of methods for entering a hypnotic trance; what's "best" is a matter of personal style and taste. Here is one procedure I teach my patients. Add whatever customizing will make the process more comfortable, as you mobilize abilities already within you.

Exercises in Self-Hypnosis

Find a quiet place where you won't be distracted. Sit comfortably in a chair with arms: feet flat on the floor, arms on the arms of the chair. Loosen clothing if you wish; take off your glasses. Remove contact lenses if they make it hard to keep your eyes closed comfortably.

Take a deep breath, and focus on how comfortably the chair supports your body. Roll your eyes upward for a moment, looking toward the center of your forehead. Let your eyelids drift downward, closing your eyes. Relax your eyes.

Now let a sense of relaxation flow down from your eyes into the rest of your face. Picture it as a thick, soothing liquid, a relaxing syrup. Let it flow down through each body part, into your arms; down through your chest, your stomach; feel it gradually fill your legs. Feel how each body part loosens, relaxes as the soothing liquid fills it.

Take a moment to feel your breathing grow deeper, slower, more even and relaxed. Let yourself become aware of the blood that flows smoothly and evenly throughout your body. Feel how limber and relaxed your muscles have become.

You may have distracting thoughts. Don't fight them or push them out of mind. Just let them pass by and float off into the background. If you hear car horns out in the street, just remember: they have nothing to do with you.

When you're ready, let yourself drift deeper and deeper into relaxation. You're entering a special protected place within your own mind. You're extremely relaxed yet highly alert. Feel pride in tapping an ability that you've had within you all your life, but perhaps are only just now discovering.

Be aware of your breathing. Use each in and out breath to pace the exercise: with each breath breathe out worry, fatigue, and self-doubt; breathe in energy, confidence, and life.

Your whole body feels pleasantly light, filled with a drifting gliding sensation. (If some image captures that for you, stay with it: perhaps a seagull soaring or a small cloud hovering weightlessly at the height of a summer sky).

After remaining in this state for a comfortable period (try ten or fifteen minutes: you may peek at the clock, but don't use an alarm), return slowly to ordinary life. One way to return is to count backward slowly from five, opening your eyes at three and reaching ordinary consciousness at one. As you do, you remind yourself that even after usual sensations return, the relaxation and its emotional benefits will continue to resonate beneath the surface of your mind. Most people like to keep activities low-key for a few more minutes before they get back into the full swing of life.

You can vary the exercise to fit your particular tastes and feelings. If relaxation seems to flow more naturally from your toes to your head than vice versa, have that thick, relaxing fluid flow uphill. If you envision relaxation as a thick, moist, warm, fragrant vapor that fills your limbs and body, by all means let it happen that way.

Once you've practiced relaxation, it's time to go a step further, with an exercise that will dramatize your ability to change your perceptions of your body. While you're deeply relaxed, try to concentrate the sense of lightness in one arm, imagining it flowing into your hand, wrist, and forearm. Feel the tingling in your hand, or some barely perceptible movement in your fingertips, and the subtle, insistent tug of a helium balloon that's attached by a cord to your wrist. Give in as it slowly, relentlessly draws your arm up. Become aware of the contrast with your other arm. If you wish, reach over and lift your "light" arm, letting it continue to float after you let go. Then imagine the helium balloon released, floating up into space as your hand slowly drifts downward.

Deep relaxation may feel more like heaviness than lightness to you. So instead of floating, let your body grow extremely heavy and perhaps warm as you relax completely. Feel your limbs turn to lead. Become aware of how solidly you're grounded in your chair, how firmly your feet are rooted on the ground.

Most important with this procedure, as with the Benson relaxation exercise, is a spectator's attitude. You're not the producer, director, actor, or critic: you simply start the procedure and observe what it's like for you. You're not *making* yourself enter a trance—you're *letting* it happen.

Whatever happens is right for you at this time. Most of us tend to monitor and evaluate our achievements: in doing the relaxation exercises, we ask, "Am I doing it right?" We question whether we feel relaxed *enough*, whether we're getting authentic results or merely deluding ourselves.

I can't emphasize too much that this line of self-doubt is not only unhelpful, it's a kind of sabotage. Self-consciousness is the enemy of relaxation. The "right" results are what *you* get—some people feel spacy, profoundly different from the way they feel before and after the exercise; others only experience a pleasantly lazy interlude. It's never been shown that a deeper, more spectacular trance state is the only path to good results. People who never get beyond relaxation may get profound benefits for their skin.

The experience may differ from one time to another, but try not to compare or rate them. As a spectator, it's not for you to give yourself marks. Don't fight natural impulses to fidget or shift around—the idea isn't to attain an unnatural position of immobility and hold it. If you feel an urge to fidget, fidget. Change your posture to make yourself more comfortable. If your nose itches, scratch it.

Because individual differences are so important, I hesitate to prescribe a "routine" of relaxation. To give it a fair chance, however, you should do one or the other exercise one to three times daily. Build it into your daily schedule—when you first get up, just before sleeping, or any time in between. If like most people you find relaxation highly pleasurable, it shouldn't be hard to keep going once you develop the habit.

Individual experiences vary widely, but many of my patients notice benefits as soon as they start doing regular relaxation: a surge of energy, a subtle but substantial change in feelings about themselves. Some find it easier to face daily hassles; they're able to put in perspective the things that once drove them up the wall. Others find it helps them get to sleep, and to enjoy deeper, more satisfying sleep. Other ways of "being good to yourself"—exercise, recreation—may come more naturally once you get the habit of giving yourself relaxation breaks.

Just one word of caution, which is necessary only when the exercise is working very well. Don't assume that because three daily sessions is good, more will be better. It may be tempting to use the safe, gratifying relaxation state as a refuge. This is better than seeking shelter in a bottle of pills or alcohol, but it's still a diversion from the business of real life. An excess of relaxation isn't "harmful" in the usual way—it won't drive you over the edge to a breakdown or render you a vegetable—but it's an escape from the serious realities that deserve our attention.

Relaxation is a thoroughly safe procedure, without side effects or pitfalls. Some people are occasionally distressed by thoughts and feelings that drift over them while deeply relaxed. Why do you feel waves of sad, happy, or anxious feelings? The healing state brings you into contact with usually inaccessible parts of your mind, the buried needs and fears of your inner self. This is nothing to worry about: you won't experience any thoughts or feelings that you aren't ready for. In fact, such feelings may be just the ones that, unfelt, have been expressing themselves in skin language. This is why I suggest that you mentally note (if you can do so without breaking your relaxation) unusual thoughts and feelings that arise as you practice these exercises.

In chapters to come, you're going to use the healing state to strengthen this direct line to your inner self. I'll prescribe exercises to continue the diagnostic work of Part I, bringing buried needs, fears, and emotional tasks within reach, so you can loosen their hold over you.

In the healing state, your mind is exceptionally open to learning. This is why certain difficult kinds of learning—breaking habits such as smoking—are often best done under hypnosis. Future chapters will give you exercises that will teach you to control your own body to reverse the processes that worsen your skin symptoms. The Eastern mystics who can raise their skin temperature by 15 degrees have learned to focus their consciousness to an incredible degree. We're only striving for a small part of their achievement.

Customizing Your Exercise

The two techniques I've described work for most people but not everyone. If you find it hard to sit motionless for fifteen minutes, go through the same motions standing up or lying down (as long as you don't fall asleep). If you can't keep your eyes closed for that long, follow the steps of either exercise while gazing out the window.

If neither exercise works for you, even with modifications to make them maximally comfortable, don't give up. Remember how various versions of the healing state are fleeting parts of all our days? You can construct your own exercise around those times when you *spontaneously* slip into this state. As you grow familiar with the healing state and the ways to get there, the confidence and energy you gain may enable you to go further with the formal exercises. If not, the benefits of the altered state gained by any means are quite real.

One of my patients, a mother of two teenagers, suffered from alopecia; after an intense personal loss, all the hair on her head and body fell out. In therapy, we gradually connected Sharon W.'s problem with the losses that ravaged her early life: the grandmother who cared for her while her mother worked would regularly pack up her bags when angry, performing a most convincing pantomime of abandonment. The first of several episodes of alopecia was triggered by the cancer and death of a close, supportive male friend. (*His* hair had fallen out because of chemotherapy.)

Sharon was uncomfortable with standard relaxation techniques, particularly with the loss of visual contact that came when she shut her eyes. So I had her sit and focus on the pleasing curve of a plant in my office, and to practice the procedure with a plant at home. She went through the same self-hypnosis technique she'd been unable to do with eyes closed. As she relaxed, she entered a kind of plant meditation, imagining the roots of the plant in their similarity to the roots of her hair, thinking of how plants and trees remain rooted despite storms, and how her hair might grow stronger and more firmly rooted, so it too could survive the emotional storms of her life.

Starting the exercise apparently helped stop the hair-loss cycle after only some head hair and one eyebrow was lost. Sharon also gained from discovering and developing her power to inhabit a special place within her own mind—unshakably *hers*, and not vulnerable to loss.

My friends who knit or crochet assure me that such needlework is a highly relaxing—one even called it hypnotic—pleasure. So I was not surprised when another patient, Nancy G., built a successful healing-state routine around the knitting she enjoyed. Nancy had a problem with scratching, so the knitting needles served the immediate purpose of keeping her hands otherwise occupied. The rhythmic motion was regular and automatic enough to allow her to focus on her breathing, to feel relaxation spreading down through her body.

As Nancy knit, she allowed her mind to drift over a skein of associations—how the wool she knit was a part of nature, how it came from sheep who cropped grass; how she was turning this wool into clothing that would keep a loved one warm; how one day when it had been patched and worn beyond repair, it might be returned to the soil, from which grass would grow for the next generation of sheep. It opened a larger consciousness that took her far from the pressures and frustrations of mundane life—indeed a restorative mental vacation.

Any number of life's activities may be your entrance into the healing state. An activity that involves rhythmical motion, like knitting, may have the same effect as repeating the word "one" in the Benson technique, or focusing on regular breathing. If you enjoy rocking in a chair, this may be the best setting for your relaxation exercise.

When your body is at rest and removed from the normal stream of stimulation, you may slip naturally into the altered state. If you're a fan of long, hot baths or showers, become aware of the special state of mind that comes over you as the minutes pass. Hot water adds a physical relaxation bonus—at around 100 degrees, your muscles loosen (this accounts for the popularity of hot tubs, jacuzzis, and saunas).

The half hour or hour you spend on the bus or train or in a car on your way to work is often a time of dulled monotony: your eyes glaze against a well-worn landscape and your mind wanders. For many people this is the beginning of the healing state, and can be deepened and used more fully.

(But *not* if you're driving!)

At the other extreme, increased stimulation may open the door. Listening to music intently (or staring intently out the window) puts your mind in a state of high alert that shifts perspective from the usual vaguely-aware-of-everything. Once you attain this focused consciousness you may be able to ease it into the healing state, using the self-hypnosis procedure.

Many people have noted the pleasurable state of mind that comes with running, biking, or any sustained strenuous exercise. Here, the rhythm of the exercise lifts you out of your normal state of mind; biochemical changes, including an increase in substances called endorphins, may also play a role.

The secret is becoming *aware* of the natural shift in attentiveness and consciousness that accompanies your regular workout, perhaps deepening it with some techniques from the formal relaxation exercises. As you run, for example, you might concentrate on your breathing, or the one-two rhythm of your stride. As you soak in the tub, allow yourself to go further and further into the dreamy, otherworldly state by focusing on your descent into deep muscular and emotional relaxation.

The goal here is developing a technique that works for you. It may not yield all the dividends of the standard exercises—you can't relax physically while you're running, and on the commuter bus it's impossible to give yourself entirely over to your inner state. But these can serve as a bridge from your regular life and consciousness to a new place within yourself you're learning to inhabit.

The important this is to *do* it—at whatever level you're ready for right now. As long as you're working on *some* healing-state exercise regularly, details aren't critical. If you find you're always interrupted, always falling asleep, or never finding the time to do it, you're on the wrong track. Try a different setting, time, or procedure—one that you'll be able to follow regularly.

It may be that despite your fine-tuning and adjustment, you somehow can't get into a healing-state habit. This may point to an emotional block or resistance to treatment that's getting in your way. We'll deal with this in a later chapter.

If you do practice the healing state regularly, you'll find it a growing source of comfort and support, whose benefits extend beyond the time you devote to it. Very likely, you'll look forward to the exercise the way we look forward to any soothing time out in the course of a busy day. In times when stress or skin troubles seem particularly severe, extra "doses" of the healing state may pay extra dividends. It's a place where wonderful things can happen, and in chapters to come we'll explore these possibilities.

12

The Ideal Imaginary Environment: A Health Spa for Your Skin

In earlier chapters, we described how emotions affect our bodies—how anger accelerates the pulse and raises blood pressure, for example. Where do they come from? We don't just react to the world out there, but to its image and echoes in our heads. The rudest postal clerk in the country can't *make* you mad. What makes you mad are the thoughts, memories, and images his or her rudeness conjures up in your mind.

You can even have the emotions and the body response without any external stimulus. Imagine, for example, that you're in bed with the sexiest movie star you can think of—or with the good-looking man or woman next door. Imagine the first kiss, the touch of skin . . . your body will go through the same process of physical arousal that would happen if you were in the real-life situation. There are people who can actually bring themselves to orgasm through the sheer power of fantasy.

If you're not in the mood for love, how about a snack—pecan pie with whipped cream? Or your favorite entree—steak, or linguine al pesto? Imagine how it looks, tastes, smells. If your mouth is watering now, all through your body glands are secreting, blood flow is shifting, muscles are readying for action. Physiologically, the thought of food calls forth a similar response to the food itself.

The power of positive thinking is no myth. Unfortunately,

the same goes for negative thinking. When we replay or antici-
pate upsetting events and encounters, we extend their stress,
multiplying the wear and tear on our bodies. When your mind
goes over yesterday's exasperating confrontation with that nasty
postal employee, your blood pressure will rise just as it did yesterday. Thoughts can kill, as dramatically demonstrated in the
"voodoo death" observed in some cultures: the victim, convinced
he is marked for death, suffers cardiac failure brought on by his
own overwhelming fears. In a far more subtle way, the needs and
fears kept alive in undone emotional tasks are an internal reality
that constantly influences physiology. They add emotions that
color each confrontation and interaction—and these translate into
harmful bodily responses.[1]

What we're attempting in this chapter is the same idea in reverse: helping you learn to manipulate your physiology in positive ways through your imagination. By taking conscious control
of a natural process, the creation of images in your mind, you
can make significant progress in becoming what you want to be:
a person with healthier skin.

The three exercises here have something important in common: in each *you imagine things the way you want them to be.* They're
a sophisticated kind of positive thinking, made deeper and more
effective by your ability to mobilize mental forces through the
healing state. In each exercise, the focused attention of the healing state deepens your bodily reaction to thoughts and feelings—
strengthening physiological changes that lead toward healthier skin.
The images of health and well-being you learn to practice here
can be self-fulfilling prophecies.

EXERCISE 1: IDEAL WELL-BEING

Just as stress and trouble strain every system of your body, happiness is good for your health. When you feel at peace and self-
confident, when all seems right with the world, the chances are
that all is right within as well. What we're going to do is use these
pinnacles of well-being as a reservoir of good emotional and
physiological feelings.

When you are in the healing state, let your mind range over your life till it finds a time—a moment, a day, a year—when everything came together: when you felt good about being yourself, when others were loving and supportive. When your dreams, if not fulfilled, at least seemed very possible—a spring morning of your soul.

The moment of well-being means different things to different people. For some, it's the combination of a pleasant setting and a loving relationship; for others, an achievement that gave a rich sense of mastery. One of my patients chose her first job as a reporter: being paid to write gave her enormous satisfaction. Another chose the afterglow of a small dinner party, where warm, supportive conversation gave a wonderful feeling of intimacy shared with his best friend. A financial consultant went way back to his days as star of a Little League team that won the New England championship. A midwestern executive simply couldn't improve on her own living room, with soft music and soft light in the wide windows.

The important thing is to chose a time and place when you felt the warmth of good feelings about yourself and your life. Once you've found it, you can go back there whenever you like to enjoy its mental and physical benefits. Don't hesitate to embellish an already delightful moment. If your life hasn't provided the right situation, improvise: imagine what such a moment would be like, or idealize a real-life experience that came close but didn't quite ring the bell.

Sit and induce the healing state of mind, and then imagine this scene as clearly and completely as possible. Let the scene build up layer by layer: sights, sounds, the sensation of sun or breeze on your skin, the particular light, the tang of the air. Add detail to detail as the scene grows vivid. For some, the image is a tableau that replays itself like a tape loop. Others enter the scene and let it play itself out of its own accord. In any case, let your mind do it; you're simply a spectator, not the producer, director, or critic of the movie. All you have to do is watch, feel, and enjoy the benefits.

These benefits include the relaxation response. But the exercise also summons up and strengthens a wealth of good feelings about the self. Every time you revisit it, your ideal well-being moment reminds you of your possibilities—who you are at your best. In ways that scientists are just now investigating, imagining ideal well-being edges your body toward the corresponding physiological state: a healthy person with healthy skin.

EXERCISE 2: CREATING THE IDEAL IMAGINARY ENVIRONMENT

Now we're going to focus imagination power where it's needed most: your skin. Examples of how the mind can influence skin physiology abound. Some thoughts can make you blush, to take a simple example. In an ingenious demonstration, Japanese researchers led volunteers sensitive to the lacquer tree (which is similar to poison ivy) under an ordinary tree that was made up to resemble a lacquer tree. The volunteers had full-scale skin eruptions—triggered by nothing more than an image, and an expectation.[2]

In this exercise you'll imagine yourself in the environment most likely to make your skin comfortable and healthy. To begin, take some time and write down everything that makes your skin feel better and worse. Emphasize concrete things like heat, cold, sunlight, coolness, dryness, friction or a smooth surface. Think of creams, ice, warm compresses. Times, places—extend your list to psychological factors, if you wish. Your guide is your own experience: what has made your skin feel better? What has soothed it, relieved itching, eased burning and pain?

The idea is to design an environment that will combine everything that's good for your skin. A setting where all forces conspire to make your skin feel as good as possible. You may develop this ideal imaginary environment by simply adding together the things that make your skin feel good and subtracting those that make it feel bad, but most people find it profitable to let their creativity take a hand. Let the environment bubble up from the riches of your unconscious. Logic and consistency are optional. Your imaginary environment can be hot and cold at the same time, icy but warm—if this is where you imagine your skin to be most happy, so be it.

Among my patients, the single most popular imaginary en-

vironment motif has been the ocean: One woman who had plantar warts imagined wading in the cool sea on a favorite beach in
Maine; a woman with eczema imagined herself on a hot, steamy
tropical seaside. Airy images are second in popularity: many people
like to feel themselves floating free on the clouds, or soaring
through the sky like a seagull, as the cool air rushes past.

For some, the imaginary environment is a skin-soothing experience at the center of a psychologically rewarding situation.
A violinist with hand eczema imagined listening to a favorite piece
of music with her father in a pleasant rustic summer setting, and
picking up a drink in a frosty glass; the coolness of the glass, the
exaltation of the music, and the comfort of a close relationship
with her sometimes elusive father made this scene triply soothing
for her skin and herself. A young man with hives used the image
of a drizzling, humid morning in Cambridge, after he'd finished
his exams. The damp, cool air eased his skin from the outside,
as his freedom from the usual burden of anxieties and pressures
relieved the tension that often exacerbated it from within.

Remember, you are the sole expert on your ideal imaginary
environment. One does not fit all, and it's not a matter of tailor-
ing the prescription to the specific problem. A majority of people
with psoriasis, for example, find warmth and sunlight helpful,
but for the minority for whom coolness works better, the ideal
environment will be a northern pine forest, not a tropical beach.

Give your imagination free rein to invent an *ideal* environment; let it include features that don't exist in this imperfect world
(what else is imagination for?). For you, the epitome of soothing
relief may be swimming the backstroke in an Olympic-size vat of
yogurt. If cold cream makes your skin feel a little better for a
little while, perhaps some quintessential moisturizing lotion, which
concentrates five hundred bottles of water in a single vial, will
multiply the feeling.

You may want to use your experiences with medicated lotions and creams. Many people, for example, get some improvement with steroid ointments, but are concerned about side effects
and avoid using them too frequently. Your mind's "conceptual
cortisone" can become just as effective, with no side effects.

As with the ideal well-being exercise, the idea is to imagine
clearly and in as much detail as possible. Use the healing state's

power to focus your mind and turn your imaginings into vivid reality, building up the scene in layers of sight, sound, smell, tang of air, quality of light. If you're walking on a beach, make it a particular beach, whether Martha's Vineyard or Puerto Vallarta. Is it noontime sun? Late afternoon? Fresh, bright morning? T-shirt? Bikini? Nude? Whether you're walking, sitting, or lying down imagine the feeling in your muscles and joints, the body consciousness that belongs to the activity. Imagine the visceral sensation of peace or excitement that goes along with dawn in the mountains or sunset on rocks sprayed by pounding surf. This is an exercise for the poet in you.

The more real you imagine the ideal imaginary environment, the more real the physiological changes that belong to it will be. These are valuable in two ways. First is simple symptom relief. The idea of this exercise is to imagine conditions and situations that will make your skin feel better: make the itching stop, ease the burning and the pain. This relief usually lingers for well beyond the exercise time itself. But the exercise also nudges your skin's physiology toward a healthier state. A world full of things that your skin likes is also a world full of whatever your skin disease *dislikes:* an internal climate less hospitable to illness.

Very slight physiological changes can have large results. I call this the Houseplant Effect, in honor of the exquisite sensitivity displayed by many of the coleus, draconia, and dieffenbachia creatures with which we share our homes. A plant that shrivels and withers in a sunny window may do fine if you alter its living conditions slightly and put it in partial shade; another will perk up and thrive in a corner that's 5 degrees warmer (or cooler) than the corner where it seemed destined for geranium heaven.

I made the point earlier that a chronic skin problem is often a matter of delicate balance—it's a disease that never gets completely better or continually worse. Anything that will nudge the balance toward health can make a critical difference: as with a houseplant, a slight change in the physiological environment may turn the trick. The small but real bodily changes that accompany the ideal imaginary environment can make life that much less easy for the virus, bacteria, or inflammatory process that is bedeviling your skin.

There's no rigid prescription for the ideal imaginary environment. Simply enter the healing state and remain in the environment as long as it feels right—five, ten, twenty minutes. Repeat the exercise as often as you have the time and need the relief it brings. Many people find that practice brings speed and depth: the more you do the exercise, the more easily you find and enter the ideal environment. Your body becomes conditioned to the rhythm of the procedure, and will move smoothly from one step to the next.

After you've begun to feel at home in the ideal imaginary environment, you may find it possible to enter it briefly almost at will. In addition to your regular sessions, summon the image up to flash through your mind dozens of times a day whenever you need it—a healing resource of inestimable value.

An Additional Technique

Some patients have successfully used a variant of the ideal imaginary environment inspired by a technique used for pain control. Imagine your hand filled to the brim with the most healing and soothing sensations imaginable. In effect, concentrate all the best features, the most comforting feelings, of the ideal imaginary environment, distilled to their essence, and pour them into the hand. When that feeling is real and full in the hand, pass it lightly over troubled areas of your skin. Imagine the healing, soothing sensation pouring forth from your fingertips, suffusing and flowing over them, leaving no room for itching, burning, or pain. When the healing sensations begin to run out, simply withdraw the hand for a few moments, let it fill up again, and then replace it on the affected area for renewed relief.[3]

EXERCISE 3: THE CELLULAR BATTLE

Your skin disorder can be thought of as a battle: virus or bacteria against your body's immune system (as in herpes, shingles, and warts) or simply the forces of health against whatever it is that is disrupting your body's natural good order. In this last "self-fulfilling prophecy" exercise, you will visualize the forces of health themselves, right among the cells, and encourage them by *imag-*

ining them overcoming whatever foreign agent or disordered process is causing your skin grief.

For inspiration, consider work that has been done in recent years with cancer patients. Pioneering doctors such as O. Carl Simonton in Texas guide their patients to imagine the struggle that is taking place between cancer cells and their bodies' defense forces. The patients are encouraged to personalize the struggle—to come up with meaningful images of cancer cells and the immune cells and other forces that oppose them: white knights against gray, greasy goblins, for example. In theory, imagining the power and potency of the body's defenses, victorious, may strengthen the forces of health, much as grief and depression weaken immune functions.[4]

I've used a similar technique with my herpes patients. Herpes recurrences reflect a struggle between a virus and the immune system. When the immune system is stronger, the virus is kept in its place; when the virus gets the upper hand, it comes out of its hiding places and erupts into an active lesion. (The same process occurs in shingles and warts.)

I ask my herpes patients to imagine what the struggle looks like: what the herpes virus is like, to them, and what kinds of forces oppose them. Using the focused power of the healing state, they image the battle with the forces of health victorious.

Images on the cellular level are as personal as the well-being and ideal-environment images. A professor saw the virus as little asterisks, and his body washing them away like a fire hydrant, with a gush of water. A dress designer saw the virus as long fish, and the body's defenses as swordfish that swim up alongside and skewer them. To an artist, the virus was black and brittle, like freeze-dried coffee, to be burned by his body and flushed away.

The essential process is making the struggle real and finding a way to participate in it actively to aid your own body in getting well. Your body's drive toward life and health is mysterious—no one knows exactly what the forces are and how they work. Here is a way to make them concrete and encourage them.

This exercise may be applied to any skin problem. It helps to have a notion of the physiology of the disease—knowing just what is or may be going wrong helps you envision your body's efforts to stop the process and correct the disorder. Psoriasis, for example, involves the rapid growth of cells that come to the surface of the skin before they're fully mature. One patient imagined them being "half-cooked" and served up by a short-order cook under pressure from his boss. His healing image was simply a more understanding boss, who encouraged the cook to slow down.

A woman with hyperhidrosis—excessive perspiration—imagined a small, lovable cleaning woman with a mop, who relentlessly mopped up excess perspiration inside the cells themselves, leaving her skin clean and dry.

A patient with recurrent skin infections imagined each one as the wound of an arrow, then imaged a transparent shield between her skin and the slings and arrows of daily life. Everything shot at her bounced off the shield. The shield had an added psychological meaning: while she was growing up, her often sadistic parents continually shot verbal and physical abuse at her.

Your images can be as close or as far from physiological reality (as you understand it) as you wish, as long as they are a personally meaningful way to make the struggle concrete and tilt it into your favor. A scientifically inclined person may image viruses as they appeared in his college biology textbook, with anatomically correct lymphocytes their conquering enemy. A more mathematical imagination may see the viruses as polyhedral soccer balls, to be deflated by a man with a needle. You may contrive a full-scale drama with little people dressed up as cells and body parts, à la Woody Allen's *Everything You Always Wanted to Know About Sex*. In any case, keep in mind how powerful your body's healthful forces are—remember how they routinely protect you from all manner of viruses and bacteria that thickly inhabit the world we live in. Aid this already powerful system by imaging allies that you endow with everything you consider strongest and most powerful in your self. Concentrate the power you already have, and bring it to bear in the struggle.

INTEGRATING THE EXERCISES INTO YOUR SELF-TREATMENT

This group of exercises is probably the most useful and powerful in the book—I've used the ideal imaginary environment, in particular, with just about all my patients, with a wealth of results both in immediate relief of symptoms and gradual improvements leading to skin health. But their very simplicity carries some dangers. They are meant to be done seriously, in an integrated self-treatment program which also includes the diagnostic work of the earlier chapters. It's easy to go through a superficial version of these imaging exercises; then if they don't work (as they very well won't, done in this spirit) the natural response is to shrug your shoulders and give up. This sabotages the whole effort, wasting a potentially valuable source of relief. Remember that the same psychological forces that may have kept your skin problem hanging on will also work underground to keep you from overcoming it. This is why I urge you to ante up the energy to work on the earlier chapters, uprooting negative images at the same time that you're replacing them with these carefully chosen positive ones.

These exercises themselves sometimes add valuable diagnostic information: your images may supply useful insights into the roots of your symptom. One woman troubled by severe scratching created an ideal imaginary environment between cool, crisp bedsheets, which suggested underlying sexual problems she hadn't realized were involved. When asked to image the struggle between herpes and her body, another woman imagined putting the virus on the plane to Europe—a way to "get rid of it" certainly, but an extremely nonaggressive mode of battle. Her choice suggested discomfort with the idea of fighting and winning—an overly conciliatory attitude that had taken its toll on more than her skin.

Often, the cellular battle exercise reveals self-sabotage that short-circuits attempts to get better. If you only see your body's good guys holding their own, not winning—or if the bad guys actually win—it's time to stop and wonder why. Likewise if you choose images that make victory all but impossible—seeing the problem as a swarm of mosquitoes and the body's defense as hands swatting them, for example.

These exercises are based on the power of belief, but it's difficult to believe they'll work until you've seen some results. Self-doubt will creep in as you learn this unfamiliar process, and healthy skepticism is only realistic. As you learn to coordinate parts of yourself you've never used before, there's bound to be a discouraging period when nothing comes together. Imaging is a skill; like playing the piano or windsurfing, it improves with practice. If you haven't felt a bit foolish at times, you're playing it too safe. If you haven't quit in discouragement, then started over a few times, you haven't really started.

If there's a single key to making these techniques work, it's making sure they don't *become work*. Keep your eye on their gamelike quality. They're a productive grown-up version of "Let's pretend," and they shouldn't be drudgery or a struggle. They're not a prescription to be swallowed, not an exercise to do for me, your dermatologist, or your family, but something soothing and enhancing to do for yourself.

13

Reinforcements: More Techniques to Help Now

The four techniques I've just described—the healing state in Chapter 11 and the three ideal imaginary environment exercises in Chapter 12—are the backbone of my program. Most people find these the most helpful against skin symptoms. But because it's a difficult, ever-changing adventure, different for everyone, I'm going to augment the basic tools with replacements and reinforcements. Depending on your personal style and needs, you may find that one or more of these extra exercises will work particularly well, on a regular basis or for an extra boost over obstacles and rough spots.

Some of these techniques are best done in the healing state, as a supplement to the basic four exercises. Others can be done at odd moments throughout the day when you need extra help.

SHORTHAND RELAXATION

The full-scale relaxation techniques described earlier have physiological benefits that extend beyond the ten or twenty minutes that you practice them. The relief you experience during the exercise itself will cast a soothing shadow into the rest of the day.

But there are times when your skin needs emergency help: when tensions mount and you feel the anxieties of life turning into eruptions. With this capsule procedure, you can bring the benefits of relaxation to the moments when you need them most.

After you've practiced the relaxation procedure for some time, your body becomes used to its sequence of physiological and mental events. You've learned the *relaxation habit*, and as with most habits you can initiate the full chain of events with a few simple cues. If you use a relaxation exercise that involves closing your eyes and feeling lightness concentrated in your right hand, for example, simply lift your right hand and touch it to your right eyebrow. Close your eyes briefly in a prolonged blink, reminding yourself of the eye closure that begins relaxation. Take a deep breath and let it out slowly, and feel relaxation flow down through your body.

Possibly the best way to develop this shorthand relaxation technique is to practice it while in the healing state. Experience how effective it can be, then keep it in reserve for when you really need it.

DISSOCIATION TECHNIQUES

Rare is the skin condition whose torment is purely physical; most people can't help compounding the agony with feelings of shame, guilt, anger, and helplessness—they develop an aggravating, punishing *relationship* with their symptoms, and as in many difficult relationships, they can gain insight and even plant the roots of lasting improvement by changing perspective—in this case, by putting some distance between themselves and their troubled skin.

The human mind has the capacity to achieve just this kind of valuable detachment. A characteristic of certain altered states of consciousness is *dissociation*—a temporary reshuffling of relations between mind, emotions, and body. This may be highly dramatic, such as the "out of the body experience" many undergo when close to death or on drug trips, but they are also commonplace and normal, occurring in the course of the average day when we focus our attention strongly on a task or on absorbing reading matter. What we experience when great art or music "takes us out of ourselves" is another familiar kind of dissocation.

Dissociation in Time and Space

In the healing state, form an intense image of yourself in the future—a person with clear, comfortable skin. Your problems are totally under control and you're thoroughly enjoying life. From this vantage point, *look back on yourself* as you now are, suffering with your troubled skin. These bad old days may be hard to remember from the perspective of the healed, healthy new you—they're just a memory now, no longer relevant to the life you lead.

Stroll casually through the experience, with no particular goal in mind: you're just reminiscing about the past. Healthy you is a sympathetic onlooker, not callous or detached from suffering you, but not emotionally involved either. When you feel like thinking about something else, just return to the healing state and life in the present.

You may find it easier to detach yourself from your symptom in space, rather than time. If the symptom is limited to a single part of your body, imagine that afflicted part floating away from you, across the room. Now it's in its normal place, now it gradually rises—a centimeter, an inch—now it floats away to a comfortable distance.

Now contemplate your arm, shoulder, leg, or whatever off in the corner of the room. That poor hunk of flesh is surely suffering and you're sympathetic. But this suffering has no direct impact on you. It's like reading a newspaper story about a typhoon that killed five hundred people in a distant, exotic land. You feel sorry for the victims, but in a fundamental sense the suffering is not yours. It has an abstract quality.

If your skin symptoms are widespread, you can carry this dissociation further. While you sit in your chair in the healing state, you divide in two. Your second self gradually frees itself from its fleshly bonds and rises, disengaged, to float up around the ceiling (you've probably seen such things in movies). As this second self, you have no skin problem: you simply float there, comfortably observing that poor tormented person with troubled skin down there in the chair.

Occasional or regular periods of dissociation give you a break, a brief time out of your troubled skin. With practice, some patients find this respite vivid and effective; they return to their regular selves with renewed resources. It's like the refreshed renewal that follows a good vacation.

Many people learn to change their relationship to their skin symptoms by taking an *emotional* step back from the events that aggravate them. The woman whose badgering husband is a regular source of distress might learn to detach and watch herself as she reacts to his provocation—as her blood pressure rises and her skin begins to burn. The anger and pain are the same, but it's almost as if someone else is enduring it. Often the ability to see such reactions with detachment is a major step toward changing them.

Anxious, hovering attention often heightens a symptom's impact and even makes it physically worse. Seeing your skin problem as a sympathetic observer would—a torment, but no curse or punishment—may break this cycle and loosen its grip on you.

In the diagnostic section of the book, I emphasized that the self has many parts. One part of you may desperately want your skin to clear, but another part has a stake in keeping your symptom holding on. And while the emotional tasks under your skin may be utterly mysterious to your conscious self, this other part of you knows what's wrong and what must be done to make your skin and your life better. *The knowledge is already there*; you are both the seeker and the hider. Here, the process of dissociation can put you in touch with knowledge to guide your efforts at self-help.

THE TALKING SYMPTOM

Your symptom and the part of the body where it resides may be expressing important emotional messages in a concrete kind of body language. Imagine the symptom as an entity with a life, personality, and experience of its own, get to understand its message better, and you will find yourself in an effective position to negotiate its departure.

This exercise is simplest when the symptom concentrates on one or several parts of the body. In the healing state, let your mind form a personified image of the afflicted part—it can be realistic, a cartoon, or a little person or an animal that for you incarnates the nature and quality of that part. If you suffer from plantar warts or eczema of the feet, for example, let your mind form a talking—perhaps dancing—foot, which may appear on the screen of consciousness with important things to say about its—and your—life and problems.

Develop a dialogue with the talking foot, arm, or generalized symptom. Take it step by step—the image may form and deepen over several days of successive practice before any conversation at all is possible. Then, as in any relationship, don't rush things with heavy disclosures and the demand for premature revelations. Start with small talk—about the weather, the Yankees. "How do the shoes feel?" "Are you tired after this long day?" Only then—after you've established the familiarity that makes trust possible—might you begin to edge into more substantive matters—how it's felt, for example, to bear the symptom.

As your relationship deepens over days and weeks, your feet may start opening up: perhaps telling you, for example, how the warts are painful, but what really scares them is getting stuck in the mud unable to walk away. They may explain the link between illness and emotion in their own "foot logic"—how the pain of the warts guarantees they'll never stay put in one place long enough to get stuck.

At a certain point, you may ask your feet what you can do to help: once their needs are out in the open, you can negotiate around them. Perhaps you can suggest a deal: you'll promise to make sure they don't get stuck in anything that frightens them; will they let go of the symptom that's been doing that job? It may be fruitful to ask your feet for their input: how can they—and you—maintain mobility and freedom in another way?

A number of my patients have gained valuable insights and made important progress this way. One man with widespread eczema initiated conversations with a ghostly, humanoid shape, the embodiment of his tormented skin. "Don't let them walk all over you," it told him. "Stand up for yourself and do your yelling and screaming verbally—not through me." Another patient with recurrent herpes gradually worked into a dialogue with the lesions, about the emotional task they had taken on. "Make sure you don't screw around, chasing after momentary pleasures, using sex as a substitute for intimacy," they told him. "You must deal with relationships seriously and in depth."

The kind of advice and information you get from your talking symptom may not be as detailed and dramatic—but trust it, and your inner self, to give you what *you* need at this particular time. Often the most important words from within are simply wise, supportive guides for living, the kind of advice we get from concerned, sympathetic friends. Among the most frequent messages are: "Take it easy," "Trust yourself," "Be honest with yourself and others about how you feel."

THE INNER ADVISER

This technique is a modern adaptation of an ancient meditation practice. It has been used widely on the West Coast by such doctors as Irving Oyle,[1] David Bresler,[2] and Martin Rossman. Here, you summon up a wise figure—perhaps a sagacious old man or woman, or a talking animal—who will help you understand the roots of your skin problem and aid your efforts to resolve it. This creature is, of course, part of yourself: the intuitive, insightful part that holds knowledge you've been unable or unwilling to articulate.

The healing state is again the door to this valuable corner of your mind. Begin by placing yourself in a calm, comfortable atmosphere—perhaps the woods or seashore of your ideal imaginary environment. Wait for a figure to appear. Perhaps a squirrel will scamper into view, or a porpoise will swim up out of the waves, or a dignified old man with a white beard will walk up and sit down next to you. Ask his or her name. It may take a number of sessions for the adviser to appear or to become familiar enough to talk with you.

The relationship can't be rushed. Gradually, in your own time—and your adviser's—you may begin to converse about your skin symptoms and your emotional tasks. As you get to know each other better, ask why you're having such problems and what you can do about them. This creature from your inner self knows much, and given the opportunity will share its knowledge with you.

A variation of the Inner Adviser technique was responsible for an important breakthrough for Dan G., the young contractor with severe warts whose case was discussed in Chapter 9. Even though his warts were no longer painful, they refused to disappear from his hands. For a year of therapy we wrestled to discover the emotional tasks that kept them holding on.

Under hypnosis, Dan visualized his hand as a bombed-out battlefield, full of craters, mounds, and seared terrain. He imagined then a construction crew whose job was to repair the damage. Over the course of several sessions Dan talked with members of the crew, asking them what was holding up progress. Was it a problem they had among themselves? Was it the working conditions? Finally, one member of the crew opened up and revealed the secret: if they repaired the pits and craters, giving Dan healthy skin, he'd have to confront the issue of going out with women—an area of his life that had long caused profound anxiety. With this in the open, it became possible to strike a bargain with the work crew: if they got on with the job of repairing his skin, Dan and I wouldn't tackle the relationship problem until he was ready. Freed from the emotional task that had shackled them, the construction crew—Dan's own forces of health—made swift progress.

This sort of interior dialogue, whether with your symptom itself, the afflicted body part, or an Inner Adviser, can become an invaluable resource. You now have a consultant or coach to help you plan and implement your therapy. Which exercises will be most helpful for you at this time? Should you spend more time in deep relaxation, or concentrate on the ideal imaginary environment? What practical changes in your work or relationships will take the pressure off your skin? The answers are already within you, but perhaps on an intuitive level that is hard to reach. These exercises simply put you in touch with the elusive part of yourself that knows so much, enlisting it as a staunch adviser and advocate in the struggle to get well.

USING YOUR INSIGHTS

As I stressed in the diagnostic section of the book, unearthing, confronting, and understanding the emotional tasks involved in your symptom is a large step in the direction of healthy skin. Here are several exercises to catalyze the process of turning insight into health.

What If It Got Better?

The healing state can help you use the "What if it got better?" exercise to explore your hidden stake in your symptom, and also provide a sustaining image of health to strive for, perhaps a self-fulfilling prophecy. After entering the healing state, imagine yourself in the future with a clear, comfortable skin. Let this image become as vivid and intense as possible. Experience this new state of health in your muscles, your blood, your skin. Enjoy a sense of freedom, of pride in all you have accomplished by courage and hard work. Fill in whatever details make the image supremely real to you: the reactions of others, the activities that you are now able to enjoy. You may want to make satisfied goals a part of the picture: imagine yourself in gratifying relationships that will make you happy; imagine your work and personal life free from wearying anxiety, full of self-confidence.

If you can imagine your health, pride, mastery, and satisfaction vividly enough, you can bring some of these positive feelings back with you. It's like borrowing on future earnings to gain benefits now. Let some of this healthy future become part of your present self.

Some of my patients worry that this exercise will feel like salt in the wound. "It's bad enough to have rotten skin," one said. "Must I torture myself with a vision of what I don't have?" You can avoid this pitfall if you affirm strongly to yourself that this is no idle dream but your *own* future, something to look forward to. Being there in fantasy is the next thing to being there in fact.

Be alert to feelings of anxiety that surface while you do this exercise. Don't ignore them, but recognize them as possible obstacles in your road to health, which you must know better in order to dispel. The more familiar you become with these anxieties, the better you'll learn where they're coming from. Repeated exposure means *desensitization:* as you learn to live more closely with these anxieties, they lose their power over you and become simple shadows instead of menacing ghosts.

Advantages of Your Symptoms

If you've used the exercise of Chapter 8 to list the hidden advantages of your skin symptoms, go further to work out how to gain them at less cost to your skin. This can be approached as any logical problem, with the focused concentration of the healing state or with input from your talking symptom or Inner Adviser.

Alternative ways to satisfy the same needs may be concrete and practical. If one advantage of hand eczema was "I don't have to wash dishes," consider getting a dishwasher, or arranging to have your spouse or roommate take on the task (trade for some other household chore). The important thing is to take the advantage—frivolous as it sounds—seriously enough to make the required changes.

If an advantage was "I get attention," or "People feel concerned and sorry," think about other ways to get the encouragement and attention you need. Make your efforts toward health, rather than your illness itself, the object of attention. Share the work you're doing with friends and family: if some people fatten on misery, there are many others who are inspired by success stories.

If an advantage was "My mother has the same problem—it gives us something to talk about," it can be satisfied with substitutes: think of other shared interests you have, and make a conscious effort to bring these into play. Perhaps the more movies or bargain basements you and your mother visit together, the less "togetherness" will be demanded of your skin. Again, the secret is taking the advantage seriously enough to change your life around it.

Giving Your Symptom Away

If "expressing anger" is an important emotional task connected to your symptom (this is the single most common one the skin is called upon to undertake), you may enjoy and benefit from giving your symptom to someone more worthy. In imagination, of course! And before you quail at the nastiness of the very idea, remember that being nasty in your head harms no one in the real world. Whatever you imagine, no one will die or go to jail; no one is going to spend a second scratching or breaking out because of your fantasy. Besides, *the anger is there already*. You are simply recognizing it, and expressing it in a harmless and helpful way.

While in the healing state, imagine, as vividly as you can, yourself giving the symptom to someone who truly deserves it— perhaps the source of annoyance that makes a regular contribution to your pains. An infuriating mother-in-law? A rapacious landlord or sadistic boss? The rock guitarist down the block who cranks up his amplifier at two in the morning? Don't spare the details. Gift-wrap your symptom, if this seems the most satisfying way to do it: leave it on a doorstep, ring the bell, and run, or lie and wait in a dark alley and when your victim appears, hand it over. Let yourself relish the victim's horror and dismay. Picture your suffering victim as he realizes what you've done, with whatever embellishments will gladden your heart.

If your symptom is in part hereditary, you may well feel angry at your parent for passing it on (an unsaintly but wholly natural anger). Then give it back! At an appropriate family ceremony, perhaps, present your symptom to the mother or father who gave it to you.

Does this exercise make you uncomfortable? This in itself is a valuable insight: perhaps a general discomfort with anger has led you to let your skin experience it for you. If this exercise makes you more comfortable with the open, unabashed expression of anger in imagined revenge, it has done a good deal.

The Ultra Time Line

This exercise takes half of the Micro Time Line of Chapter 5 down to a more precise level, leaving the triggering factors and mood fluctuations for another time and concentrating on the ups and downs of the symptom itself. It particularly appeals to people who feel more comfortable with concrete numbers than with abstractions and emotions. Despite obvious differences, this exercise has much in common with techniques like dissociation: here too you gain detachment and a new awareness of your symptom.

For a week or two before you begin the treatment exercises in earnest, keep very close track of your skin condition. Five times a day (in the morning, before lunch, midafternoon, dinnertime, bedtime, perhaps) give a numerical rating to the physical and psychological aspects of your symptom. Let 100 be the worst it's ever been, 0 total cure. Take a mirror if necessary and examine your skin for three or four minutes and rate its appearance. Count the warts, pimples, or lesions. Give another rating to the physical sensations—the pain, itching, or burning—of your skin during that part of the day. A third rating should reflect the symptom's psychological impact for that period—just how much it is getting to you. If a behavior—like scratching or pulling your hair—is a part of the problem, record how often you do it.

Does your symptom arouse self-deprecatory thoughts? Record how often you give yourself a hard time with an inner monologue that keeps on repeating, "Nobody will want to go out with me," "I look like hell," and such things. A portable golf counter, worn as a wristwatch or ring and touched each time you hear yourself repeating the party line, may be most helpful.

Make a graph with three lines in different-colored inks: the appearance, the physical symptom, its emotional impact and how much it is getting to you. This will give you a graphic record of the minutest fluctuations of your symptom. Keep it up as you begin the treatment exercises, and watch for changes.

Many people are surprised to find that this sort of meticulous record keeping, in itself, brings actual improvement. Some psychologists suggest that it diverts some of the energy used in producing the symptom into recording it, or that it brings the whole symptom-producing process up to a more conscious level. One thing the Ultra Time Line gives you is the opportunity to respond actively and constructively to your symptom—something other than scratching to do with your hand. If you post your chart in a conspicuous place, like the refrigerator door, it will get other people off your back. Instead of constantly asking how you're doing, they can see for themselves. (You might suggest to friends and family at this time that you appreciate positive comments about improvements more than remarks about setbacks. Or have a rule: positive feedback only.)

Ratings by Other People

I've heard these words many times: "My friends say my skin is getting better, but I don't think so." Sometimes the owner of a skin condition is the last to notice improvements. He or she loses out on the reward, encouragement, and momentum that it should bring.

If you wonder whether this applies to you, ask an objective friend or family member to observe and rate numerically your skin condition, noting your progress as your treatment program gets underway. If there are significant discrepancies between your rating and his or hers—if you remain blind to improvements that he or she sees clearly—consider the possibility that you're sabotaging your own self-help at some level. Perhaps you should redouble your work to discover the unconscious advantages and secondary gains that keep the symptom at work, and if you are ready, seek professional help in unearthing them.

PUTTING YOURSELF IN CHARGE

A fundamental aim of this book is to give you more control over your body, your symptom in particular. The thing that many people find most distressing in persistent illness is the feeling that their bodies and their lives are not under their control; to feel yourself in the driver's seat is, in itself, an antidote for this frustration and despair.

The truth is that you're already in control of your body—a part of your mind is possibly maintaining your symptom with a kind of negative hypnosis. The following exercises will help you *feel your control*—and use it consciously for health.

Telling Your Skin What to Do

Anyone who's reared a child or raised a puppy or kitten knows that a certain amount of nagging is part of the job. You simply must remind a child or pet *not* to do the things that are not to be done: to stay away from the stove or the houseplants, to refrain from chewing on slippers. Nagging has a poor image, deservedly when it is done to excess, but actually its repetitive lessons are a vital part of the learning process.

The same approach can be surprisingly successful with many skin problems—with the symptoms themselves, as well as the repetitive thoughts and feelings that make the suffering worse. Your skin, quite possibly, is something of an unruly child, and may respond better to authoritative commands than to an excess of whining and cajolery.

When your skin starts to bother you—to itch, burn, hurt, or whatever—tell it to stop. Firmly, of course, for this will need persistent repetition; a single injunction never kept Rover out of the petunias permanently. But it may give you a brief and very welcome respite. As important, it demonstrates your power over your skin. But what you're doing here isn't a mere power trip, any more than the mother who tells her child repeatedly to stay away from the stove is exercising power for the fun of it. She—and you—are showing your love and concern by setting appropriate, protective limits. By your willingness to keep at this exercise, to remind your skin, over and over again, what it must not do, you're expressing the same caring attitude that a parent expresses when he reminds a child—for the hundredth time—not to play with matches.

You may use a similar approach when you're bedeviled by self-deprecating thoughts and anxious feelings about your skin. If you pass an attractive member of the opposite sex and hear your inner voice beginning a familiar litany—"She thinks I look like raw hamburger"—talk back to yourself, with a firm, no-nonsense "Stop!"

With yourself, as with kids and kittens, tone is the key. Some tones of voice get results, some don't. What works best is neither a namby-pamby whine nor the menacing bark of a drill sergeant. Keep in your mind the image of a firm, fair parent, as you talk turkey to the unruly child in your head, heart, or skin.

Nibbling

Every successful salesman knows this technique, as does every kid who wants something badly: get your foot in the door, and the rest will eventually follow. A journey of a thousand miles begins with a single step.

Nibbling away at your symptom is a foot-in-the-door technique. Just taking a first step establishes your ability to change your skin for the better, paving the way for a whole chain of improvements to follow.

Instead of trying to cure your symptoms all over your body, altogether, aim at first for a 10 percent improvement. If your hives seem to be everywhere, don't try to make them all go away, but concentrate on one area—your left shoulder, for example. Let that body part get all the benefit of the imaginary ideal environment. Make sure it is pampered and eased during your relaxation exercises. Visualize yourself, while in the healing state, with no hives on your left shoulder. Lower the stakes! Remind yourself that whether that single shoulder gets better or not doesn't really matter—you're not staking much on the outcome.

Use a similar technique with skin problems that recur periodically. If you have herpes outbreaks monthly, forget about getting rid of them altogether, for now, and make your first goal skipping a month, or lengthening the healthy interval to six weeks. If your episodes always last seven days, work on cutting them down to six.

The same sneaky persistence may help you deal better with the factors that trigger your skin eruptions. Has it become clear that certain situations and encounters give your skin a particular beating? Suppose, for example, that your skin suffers every time your parents nag you as if you were still a small child. First imagine the 100 percent full-scale attack that's guaranteed to trigger your symptoms: the time, for example, that your mother called and nagged you every day for a week. Then imagine scaled-down versions of the same irritant—a 90 percent version, an 80 percent version, and so on. What is a 10 percent version of this skin-scathing stress? Perhaps an offhand, belittling remark from your mother, which she quickly retracts.

Go through your usual healing-state exercise, and imagine yourself in the imaginary ideal environment. Think of the 10 percent aggravation—let yourself get caught up in it vividly. Then stop and relax. Return to your imaginary ideal environment; see yourself experiencing the annoying situation, but not responding to it physically. Once you've mastered the first bite of annoyance, imagine yourself in the 20 percent situation—your mother telling you to get a haircut the same way she did when you were seventeen, for example. Again, experience the situation fully in your head, but let its impact roll off your body. Tell yourself: "Okay, this is an aggravation. But I can protect my body and my skin." Don't pretend it's without pain, but try not to let it get to you. Strive for the spectator's detachment.

What you're doing is nibbling away at the triggering annoyances in your imagination—defusing them a little at a time. For this technique to work it is essential not to rush things. Write down each 10 percent, 20 percent, etc. step, and do no more than two in any one day. Do each until you can experience physical relaxation while imagining the annoyance—it's there, but it doesn't get to you. Every step in this direction makes it easier to protect your skin when the real-life situations come up: not by pretending there's no pain, but by taking control of its physiological impact.

Controlled Experiment

Scientists often compare an experimental group with a control group to measure the value of a new drug—the experimental group gets the drug, the control group doesn't. You can use the same technique to prove to yourself that your own treatment methods are working, particularly if the results are subtle and you aren't quite convinced of your ability to help your skin.

Divide your affected skin into two areas of comparable severity. Make the most troubled the experimental side, the least troubled the control. As you go through your treatment exercises, focus on the experimental side; imagine that your control side is entirely indifferent to what you're doing. As improvements occur, this method will highlight and dramatize them. And once the first side improves, you can rest assured the other side will respond to the same techniques.

Symptom Substitution

Even when the emotional issues behind a symptom are stubbornly hidden and difficult to work through, it is often possible to negotiate with them. That is, you may be able to exchange your symptom for a "counterfeit" activity that accomplishes the same emotional tasks in a benign fashion: scratching away at a violin, for example, instead of scratching your skin. W. S. Kroger, a pioneer in hypnosis, treated a woman whose persistent scratching had resisted all dermatological and psychological therapy for seven years. Over a period of two weeks, she was able to substitute scratching the "skin" of a large doll, which she kept beside her while she slept and watched television, for scratching herself.[3]

If you can't trade in your symptom for a harmless substitute, you may be able to "trade down" for a less troublesome version. Often, symptoms substitute themselves spontaneously. A person who suffers from eczema as a child may later in life enjoy clear skin, but endure persistent hay fever. The energy of needs, fears, and emotional tasks may take many paths, appearing now as symptoms in the skin, now as manifestations elsewhere.

The ability to give yourself a headache may seem a dubious power, but it is power all the same. To *exchange* your itch for a headache demonstrates your mastery of your body. Proving that the symptom is yours, substitution may take you an important first step on the road to controlling it well enough to let it go.

In the healing state, plant the suggestion that an innocuous activity will do the work of your skin symptom. When angry, you might tell yourself, you're going to chop wood, or beat carpets, or pound the pavement in a five-mile run. You will satisfy your "need" for scratching by applying sandpaper to wood. If this seems too abrupt, suggest a deal to yourself. For example, if mild headaches would be easier to bear than your chronic itch, plant the substitution suggestion. Remind yourself of it from time to time throughout the day. You may find, in fact, that your skin is better while you "pay dues" with occasional headaches.

Making Your Symptom Worse

If you remain absolutely unconvinced of your power to make your skin better and are about to add this book to your pile of rejected doctors and their remedies, I have one last challenge: can you make your symptom worse? I don't recommend this technique routinely—I save it for angry, skeptical, disgusted patients who need a last-ditch demonstration. Perverse as it sounds, a number of people have used this exercise to feel their power over their bodies. It was a first step toward applying that power for health.

Fred, for example, was a hard-nosed, logical engineer who simply could not relate to the psychodynamics of symptoms. His skin was red, raw, and itching, he firmly knew, because there was a physical problem, as a mechanical malfunction invariably reflected something physically wrong with a machine.

I challenged Fred—I told him he had the power to take any patch of skin that was clear, and make it itchy. The perversity of the idea appealed to him, and he gave it a try, and before long he became able to experience much of the same discomfort in healthy skin that he'd had in the red, raw patches. He saw for himself that the mind-body connection was real, and this was an enormous help in getting on with other techniques.

If you can make your skin worse, you can make it better. The idea is to do anything you can think of in the most negative, stress-inducing way possible, *maximizing* its adverse effect on your skin. It's a challenge—can you make your skin worse with mind power? For example, try nonrelaxation. Go down through your body, step by step, part by part, heightening feelings of tension. Imagine all your annoyances getting worse and inflicting themselves on your skin, making symptoms more severe and intense.

Place yourself in an unideal imaginary environment: summon up the worst times of your life—the times you felt most miserable and betrayed. Make a list of everything that makes your skin most uncomfortable, and construct an imaginary environment that brings all these features together. Are you fed up, disgusted, angry with the time and money you've wasted with dermatologists . . . and now with this book? Keep these angry feelings at the front of your mind as you exert all your energies in a last-ditch attempt to make it all worse.

From here it may be a short step to the beginnings of self-mastery that will make it better.

I want to stress again that this gallery of exercises is primarily for your contemplation. With the exception of the "shorthand" technique, many of my patients don't use any of them—they concentrate on the four central exercises. Virtually no one adds more than one or two to the treatment program.

You might do best simply to read about them as interesting background material—things that have worked for various people—and forget about them. If you need them, they'll probably just pop into your head at the appropriate time. Feel free to experiment with any or all of these exercises, as long as you don't fall into a dilettante approach that skips from one to another without ever getting serious about any. Whichever exercises you decide to use will require serious commitment.

Above all, don't worry about choosing the exercise that's "right for you." It's all a matter of taste and style, and it would make as much sense to worry about whether you *should* prefer chocolate or vanilla.

If you're inspired by any or all of these exercises to improvise your own technique, that might be the best choice of all.

14

Thinking:
Enemy or Ally

Throughout this book I've focused on two parts of the typical skin problem—the physical symptom itself and the feelings connected to it. But we don't just feel our problems, we also think about them. Your thoughts about your skin are too important to overlook.

This is particularly true for the many people who are more comfortable talking about thoughts than feelings. Engineers and scientists, for example, often find extended discussions of emotion mushy and imprecise; they relate more readily to logical statements that can be proved true or false.

Many people are more in touch with their thoughts than with their feelings. They don't consciously feel unloved, or guilty, or empty inside. But because they're tuned in to their thoughts about themselves and others, they can calmly, logically relate that "this herpes may hurt my odds in the marriage market." If you ask them, they'll tell you they have no feelings about this turn of events; it's just a statement of fact.

The feelings, of course, are there—somewhere. It's less painful to dwell on thoughts than to experience feelings, and people may fall into this overintellectualized habit of mind for self-protection. The tendency itself becomes painful in those who can't get thoughts out of their heads and run the same thinking tape over and over. Such people, who suffer from what psychologists call obsessional neurosis, are often highly organized and productive. Their thinking processes are admirably developed, but they run on ceaselessly with a life of their own, like a head without a horseman.[1]

Such thoughts were a big part of Charles B.'s problem. When Charles, a writer, contracted genital herpes, he entered a protracted period of moral anguish. He became obsessed with his symptom and the sense of his own badness. Unable to stop thinking of either, he endured an endless stream of self-recrimination on the subject of his low morals and the harm he might have done to women in the months before he realized that he was "contaminated." He uncontrollably moralized to himself like a relentless evangelist addressing a shameless libertine.

At one point, Charles's obsession took a bizarre turn. While listening to a radio discussion of herpes, he heard about herpes encephalitis, an *exceedingly rare* complication in which the virus attacks the brain. This is never a consequence of genital herpes. But when he shortly thereafter developed a rash on his scalp, Charles was convinced that he'd been struck by this rare, fatal infection—just deserts for his evil behavior!

In Charles's case, one hapless person harbored three illnesses. There was the physical herpes, caused by a virus; there was "psychological herpes," the self-punishing thoughts that made the physical disease an exaggerated torment; and there was a scalp rash brought on by the obsessive attention that Charles had focused on this part of his body. Charles had *thought* himself into this last illness.

In therapy, I helped Charles to look beyond the obsessional thoughts to their emotional message, which had nothing at all to do with herpes. Why did he feel himself to be such a bad person—when and how had he been brainwashed? All this difficulty and anguish, he came to realize, had begun long before he'd ever heard of herpes; the better he understood this, the more in touch he became with the feelings of badness that lay beyond the distorted thoughts ("I got herpes because I'm depraved") they engendered.

Charles did well in psychotherapy, as he learned to see the anger and sexual feelings that lay beneath his obsessive thoughts.

Similarly, he came to realize that his concerns about his brain were linked less to any real danger than to the grim reality of his father's health, whose mind was deteriorating with Alzheimer's disease.

Some therapists feel that many if not most emotional problems reflect distorted thinking patterns: depression, anxiety, and other ills, in their book, follow false ideas about oneself and the world. I believe that these distortions and painful emotions are like the head and tail of a coin.

This is particularly clear in people whose thoughts are distorted into *delusions*—they are convinced they have a disease, for example, that does not physically exist. Recently, a psychiatrist in San Francisco reported growing numbers of people who visit doctors with the conviction that they have genital herpes. There is no evidence of the disease—not even the most minute lesion, in some cases—but they are convinced. They experience the full gamut of guilt, rage, and self-blame that many authentic herpes patients endure.

The psychiatrist compared these people to those who come forth to confess whenever the papers report a grisly murder. Such imaginary murderers are obsessed with a deep sense of their own badness. They feel as if they've done something unspeakable; then when they read about the murder, they're convinced this is the unspeakable thing they've done. The delusion fits their sense of guilt.[2]

In the same way, victims of "delusionary herpes" have been convinced by exaggerated press, TV, and magazine reports that herpes is a dreadful thing, the fitting punishment for promiscuity and depravity. They *already* feel evil, and thus it is natural for them to delude themselves that they harbor the disease. If the false belief is firmly entrenched, all the dermatologists and negative lab tests in the world cannot shake it. Genital herpes is such a perfect *metaphor* for their feelings about themselves that they cannot let go.

A person with such a delusion has serious emotional problems and urgently needs professional help. The best thing anyone can do is help him to get the therapy he needs; with proper care, these disorders are often quite treatable. One thing you can't do is talk such a person out of his delusion—to argue that the "lice" that torment him are actually lint, or that the horrid rash that is taking over her entire body is invisible to everyone else. Keep in mind that the delusion itself is but the tip of the iceberg: a person who feels consumed by nonexistent disease is actually telling you he is tormented by unbearable feelings. His beliefs may be an inaccurate description of physical reality—there are no lice, no herpes lesions, no rash—but they clearly express his inner emotional anguish.[3]

In a similar if less flamboyant way, the distorted thoughts that torment many skin sufferers may express emotional realities with which they are out of touch. Thoughts like "These hives are gross—nobody wants to touch me," or "Psoriasis shows I have weak genes—I'm biologically unfit," inaccurate as they are, may point the way to important emotional truths.

Why become more aware of your distorted thinking about your skin problems? For one thing, when you tune in to the silent statements you constantly repeat to yourself, you've taken a first step toward seeing the less alarming truth. Their emotional underpinning gives these thoughts staying power—they resist the light of reason—yet many people become able to *argue* with their distortions. Challenged repeatedly, they lose some of their power to torment. For another, these automatic thoughts can be a valuable clue to the needs, fears, and tasks that lie deeply buried, particularly if you are the kind of person who is "not in touch with your feelings."

For example, a patient of mine who suffered from severe acne habitually thought to himself, as he walked down the street: "I look like hell. Nobody wants to be seen in public with me." If an attractive woman approached, Jack would flinch in anticipation, thinking, "She's going to be repulsed when she gets a look at this open sore I call my face."

There was a little truth in Jack's train of thought, but a lot of distortion. True, his face didn't look as clear as it might have, and he'd have been more attractive with better skin. But the fact was that the skin of his face was only a small portion of his total identity—a small portion, for that matter, of his total skin. The idea that onlookers were disgusted and avoided him was absolutely untrue, as he himself conceded when we compared his self-tormenting ideas with his actual experience.

Jack had been playing this tape of terrible thoughts so long that they'd become second nature. An important first step was just *becoming aware* that he'd fallen into this habit. A second step was separating feelings from facts and recognizing that in the light of logic, these beliefs were false. He gradually learned to substitute a more accurate train of thought: "My skin is not superb, but it doesn't look *that* ghastly. Plus I have a lot to offer behind my face; my friends are clearly aware of this, and it's possible to make others see it too."

Jack had found it hard, up to this time, to tune in on his feelings about himself and his skin condition. But these habitual thoughts, once recognized, provided a handle on his feelings: he came to appreciate how he tended to see things in black and white (if his skin wasn't great, it was terrible) and to come down hard on himself. He simply *felt* unworthy and unlovable, for reasons that had nothing to do with his acne. This realization began a process of changing the images and feelings that had long made Jack miserable in a way that was anything but skin deep.

Our ideas are products of our social environment: the more of a stigma a disease bears, the more difficulty it's likely to create. Thus people like Jack, whose skin problems are highly visible, have particular trouble with self-punishing thoughts. This is also one reason why people with genital herpes are so vulnerable to tormenting thought distortions: they've swallowed a steady diet of mythology that equates herpes with evil sexuality, and this has infected their ideas about themselves more than any virus.

Knowing the truth may not make you entirely free, but it can ease pain with perspective. Remember one thing: social mythology is irrational and changeable. Today there's a strong social stigma attached to lice, for example. But back in the middle ages, lice were a nuisance for lords and ladies as well as the common people, and reflected nothing on one's character, morality, upbringing, or class. But *psoriasis*—now there was a disease that marked its victims as outcasts. Why? Because it was mistakenly thought to be a close relative of leprosy, a disease with which it actually has absolutely nothing in common. Psoriatics were shunned—and no doubt thought terrible things about themselves—because of tragic misinformation.[4]

On some level, we know the truth about herpes; even in the panic that may follow the first lesion, there's a small corner of the brain that keeps these facts on file. The task is to recognize what distorted thoughts have taken over to logically combat distortion with fact, and ultimately to recognize what emotional drives give the distortion its power. This is what we will attempt in the following exercise.

Many people find this easiest with a large sheet of paper divided into three columns. Tune in to the inner monologue of thoughts about your skin. Become aware of the statements—the pseudofacts—that you habitually repeat to yourself. Jot them down in the first column. For the second column, look at these statements coolly and logically. Sum up the real facts that correct the distortions of column one. The third column is where you explain to yourself where the distortions of column one came from. This means opening yourself up to the buried feelings, needs, and fears that are expressed in your automatic thoughts.

For example, one distorted thought that commonly bedevils people with genital herpes is: "No one will want to have any relationship with me. I'll never be able to marry." In the second column, the logical refutation might go: "I will have to take precautions, and sometimes talk about my problem in a more open manner than I would otherwise, but I know that many people with herpes have good sex lives and good marriages." In column three, introspective analysis might suggest: "Before I ever heard of herpes, I was prone to self-doubt. I've long worried about my desirability, and that doubt has fastened on herpes." Anything that helps you to understand where the pseudo-conclusion of column one comes from belongs in column three. You might include the "scarlet letter" line that part of society sells about herpes.

This exercise demands logic and honesty to separate half-truths from real truths. The thought that oppresses many long-term sufferers of conditions like herpes, vitiligo, psoriasis, and alopecia is one such half-truth: "I've suffered for years and I'll suffer forever. There's no cure for my illness." The truth is that while doctors and their medical technology can't totally cure these ills, many people have gotten better spontaneously, through their bodies' own healing forces. Psoriasis is not "curable," but is treatable, and a person who goes for years with only a small patch here and there has won an important, if not total, victory. Similarly, about one-third of people with herpes suffer only a single outbreak, and then the virus retreats more or less for good to its hiding places in the nerve cells. New drugs help suppress the virus, and it is possible to live with it without pain or trouble—millions of people do. Even for those who do have continuing recurrences, each is successfully cured by the immune system. What emotional needs and tasks might make you dwell on having an incurable disease? Do you find it hard for some reason to accept the idea of curing yourself? Put the answer in column three.

Similarly, a common concern among people with chronic skin problems is: "My body's defenses are shot; there's something weak about my constitution or else the problem would not torment me. A really serious disease—cancer? AIDS?—is just around the corner." The fallacy here is apparent if you consider all the organisms and illnesses that your immune system fights off every minute of every day. And even if your warts linger or your herpes recurs regularly, most of the time your immune system is keeping the virus under control. In column three, where you dig for the roots of your thought distortions, you may note that you tend to cast things in black and white. And perhaps that your belief in the weakness of your body's defenses reflects deeper feelings of weakness and incompetence. Similar distortions may be unearthed by people with hereditary diseases, such as psoriasis, who believe that they have "tainted genes" or "bad heredity." The truth is that illness carried by one gene or gene set says nothing about the millions of other genes with which we're each endowed; the belief in poor genes, however, may say a good deal about your feelings about yourself and your parents.

Your feelings about yourself and your parents? Does that truly have at all that much to do with your skin problem? If you've read this far and still find yourself thinking under your breath, "All this sounds fine, but I know my lupus is a purely medical matter, a question of plumbing," write this in column one. In column two, you might observe (if indeed you've made the observation) that your skin does in fact improve and get worse in good times and bad times; that much evidence does, in fact, link your mind and your body. Column three? Perhaps you are frightened to think of how large a role emotions play in your life, how active your participation in your illness may be. Perhaps you find it more comfortable to see yourself as victim.

Although I hate to think of anyone's using my book this way, I can imagine any number of people reading it, shaking their heads ruefully, and saying to themselves, "This guy's telling me what I knew all along. If only I had my head on straight, I wouldn't have all this trouble. I'm a *real* loser—not only do I have this revolting skin, but I gave it to myself." If you're giving yourself this kind of hard time, try to be objective and logical in column two—write down what you'd say to a friend who came out with that sort of nonsense: "I've done the best I can to handle the stresses and conflicts in my life. I've never *consciously, intentionally* hurt myself or my skin. If I haven't been as effective as I'd like in dealing with emotional turmoil, it's not because I'm lazy, bad, or incompetent. I need new techniques and practice to get better—and I'm giving this my best shot." Remember the difference between responsibility and blame; you may be *responsible* for your skin, insofar as your emotional needs have played a significant role in it. But such needs are legitimate and beyond your control, so it is thoroughly inappropriate to *blame* yourself—as unfair as it would be to chastise a famished child for taking a mouthful of bread.

You might realize (and note in column three) that your reaction to the book reflects a general tendency to blame yourself, to attribute everything and anything to your inadequacy and weakness. Focusing on this sense of inner worthlessness could initiate a train of questions: Was I brainwashed? Who taught me to think I was a jerk? What carrot or stick did they use? By column three, the habitual self-flagellation of column one could become the kind of questioning that can change far more than your skin.[5]

15

Biofeedback: The Electronic Doctor

There are many paths to any mountaintop, including the exciting "mountaintop" we've been discussing in recent chapters—the ability to control your body for better skin health. Techniques like relaxation and self-hypnosis are two such paths.

We live in a world of machines and circuits as well as ideas and beliefs, and modern technology has cleared its own path to physiological control—biofeedback. Put most simply, biofeedback is a tool that may help you learn better control over your body.

The inspiration for biofeedback comes from the other side of the mountain—the mystical side. For years, observers have been intrigued and puzzled by the ability of Eastern mystics, such as yogis, to dramatically alter their body functions. Scientists were amazed at reports of men who could slow down their normal life processes enough to survive months of burial in airtight containers. Here was "relaxation" taken to its farthest extreme! Others, apparently, had learned to speed up their metabolism. Clad in their simple garments, monks performed one religious exercise by immersing themselves in an icy river high in the Himalayas. Three times they leaped in—and three times they dried themselves and their robes by sharply raising their body temperature, generating a sort of "psychic heat."[1]

How had the monks learned such impressive control over their bodies? The "wisdom of the ages" accumulated generations of experience, fine-tuned it, and encapsulated it in religious exercises that monks practiced over decades of committed concentration. Such long, ascetic rigors are not for most modern men and women, to be sure. To scientists, the importance of the phenomena was the assurance that *the ability was there*, in the human mind. The monks had learned to unlock it: they had proved that human beings could control what doctors and scientists had always thought involuntary body functions. And if they could do it their way, why couldn't we do it our way?

The idea of biofeedback is simple. A thermometer or other sensing device is attached to the body, where it constantly monitors a physiological factor such as body temperature, muscle tension, heart rate, or skin moisture. Lights, meter readouts, or tones that rise and fall tell you whether the dimension under study increases, decreases, or holds steady.

For example, a doctor using biofeedback may place an electrode on your forehead to monitor muscle tension. He'll say: "The tone will rise if tension increases, and lower if it drops. Try to make the tone lower." Without knowing exactly how they do it, most people learn rather quickly to lower the tone—and thus to reduce muscle tension. This has been used for effective headache therapy.

Biofeedback is essentially an aid to learning. To learn most skills, it is helpful if not essential to know how you're doing. How could you learn to throw a ball straight and true if you couldn't see where it went after you released it? When attempting to learn something as unfamiliar as relaxation or physiological control, some people find it hard to know if they're doing it right. (Is your body relaxed, or are you fooling yourself?) Like the bathroom scale that aids many in weight reduction, biofeedback tells you how you're doing.

Developing any kind of physical skill often means *discovering* how to accomplish what you want, and then trying to duplicate the accomplishment. For example, you don't know how to throw a ball well until you've done it. Others can coach you, you can read books and pick up pointers; these can show you the way, but the critical breakthrough is getting off a good throw yourself and feeling the experience in your own muscles. You throw the ball and see it go the way you want, and from then on you're trying to recapture the muscular feeling that went with the throw and practicing it until you have it by heart.

The physiological skills we're talking about here are similar. For all our hints, formulas, and suggestions on relaxation, for example, you don't know how to do it until you've done it—until you have the feeling in your body. Once you've found the way to relaxation, you're more likely to find it again. The usual way to learn relaxation or self-hypnosis is simply trying to exercise, gradually recognizing the distinctive feelings, and learning to get there with more and more assurance.

But some people may find the way elusive. They may in fact be getting there, but slowly, accomplishing changes they are unable to recognize. Biofeedback can tell them that their hand temperature is rising, or their sweat glands have slowed down (both physiological signs of relaxation). It tells them that *they're doing something right*. Even if they can't say just what they were doing, because they know how it *feels* to begin relaxing they can get there more easily and go further and deeper into the state.

Thus far, biofeedback has proved helpful in a range of disorders, including tension and migraine headaches, premenstrual cramping, Reynaud's disease, and irritable bowel syndrome. With the help of its devices, patients have learned to lower blood pressure, overcome insomnia, and manage phobias. Biofeedback has aided the relief of pain due to muscle tension in the neck and lower back.[2]

You may note that this list is similar to the health problems for which relaxation and hypnosis have been effective. They are, in fact, related to stress and the extra burden that unresolved emotional tasks impose on the body, and for which biofeedback, like the other techniques, can be an antidote.

Up till now, there has been little (surprisingly little) application of biofeedback to skin disorders: we do not yet know how useful a resource it will be. But studies suggest that some people, at least, can benefit from its technological assist. Like the exercises we've been discussing, biofeedback may help troubled skin in two ways: via relaxation and via specific physiological alterations in the troubled area. But in truth, we're still at the edge of understanding why biofeedback works for some people and not others and what it does.

For example, one research project tried biofeedback with five patients who had such severe dyshidrotic eczema (a form of eczema that produces extremely dry skin) that even potent steroid drugs couldn't give adequate relief. They were trained to relax and to raise the temperature of their hands. All the patients improved in three to six sessions, and those whose flare-ups were most closely linked to emotional turmoil did best. But there was no connection between the effectiveness of the biofeedback training—how successfully the patients learned to raise their hand temperature—and how much relief they found.[3]

Another experiment got down into the physiology of the problem. Psoriasis comes from a rapid rate of skin-cell growth, and these investigators proposed that lowered skin temperature might mean slower cell growth. Three doctors in Texas worked closely with three patients, using auditory and visual feedback: they told their patients to make the tone lower, or meter readout drop, by making their skin cooler. The drop was not dramatic— an average of 1.3°F per session. But it was enough to reduce the rate of cell production, according to skin biopsy. Improvements in the psoriasis were noticeable. However, they only lasted for four months before the original condition began to return.[4]

How does biofeedback work? Does it actually change physiology in a specific area, or produce a more general relaxation? Using biofeedback equipment promotes a state of concentration that produces deep relaxation in many people; those who are good hypnotic subjects may find themselves entering a trance or healing state. In a Dutch study, eleven of fourteen patients were able to control their hyperhidrosis—chronic excessive sweating—with the help of biofeedback. But the researchers suspected the active ingredient was actually relaxation.[5]

Would these subjects have relaxed as well—and improved as much—*without* biofeedback? This is unclear. In other studies, skin patients reported a gratifying sense of well-being and enhanced self-control with biofeedback. It put them in the driver's seat and gave them an active role in fighting their illness. As I've said often, the sense of mastery is often vital in the psychological process of getting well. But was biofeedback *necessary* to produce this?

As far as any individual is concerned, that question doesn't really matter. "If it works, do it" is the soundest advice I can give where you're fighting your own fight against an elusive enemy that no one, yourself, your doctors, or the experts, can claim to understand fully.

There are probably some people for whom biofeedback is simply a quicker way to relaxation and physiological control— the fastest path up the mountain. Who are they? Research hasn't yet shed much light on this question, but it may be those who are most at home with technology, who feel comfortable using electronic devices and like to have numbers confirm their feelings and intuitions.

It may be a matter of temperament. If you're prone to self-doubt, if you practice relaxation techniques but are plagued by the fear that nothing's really happening, the concrete readout numbers or changing tone of a biofeedback device will ease your fears and take performance pressure off. Instead of constantly asking yourself "How am I doing?" you'll have the answer right in front of you.

If you want to try biofeedback for your skin problem, remember that you're a pioneer in a territory that scientists and doctors are just beginning to explore. You yourself are going to be your own research subject. A growing number of practitioners, from technicians to trained physicians and psychologists, may be able to help you in various ways, but the chances are they haven't used biofeedback with your particular condition either, so you'll have to learn and work together. (See Appendix II for suggestions on finding professional help.)

Those who want to go it on their own can choose from a number of home biofeedback devices available for under $100. The most common are digital thermometers, some with sensors that attach to your body. Such a device needn't have bells and whistles, but it should have a continuous readout and be sensitive to differences of .1 degree.

Another device that's usually easy to find measures what's called galvanic skin response or GSR. The more your skin perspires, the better it conducts tiny amounts of electricity. Because you perspire more when you're tense and less when you're relaxed, GSR is a widely used measure of tension—it's one of the things monitored by a polygram or lie detector, for example. Also available are wristwatches that will continuously read out pulse rate (runners sometimes use them). All this equipment can best be found in a store, department, or mail-order catalog that specializes in health and stress reduction.

How can you put this equipment to work? The most effective approach may be combining biofeedback with specific techniques for relaxation, symptom relief, and imaging. This is what a psychologist at Texas State University did with a group of acne patients. They continued to use their usual medication, benzoyl peroxide; but in a state of relaxation assisted by biofeedback, they were told to visualize the medication penetrating their pores, opening up and pushing up impactions. Twenty-two patients who received this three-pronged assault of biofeedback-assisted relaxation, imaging, and medication improved 25 percent faster than those who got the medication alone.[6]

Try your own experiment. If you're working with relaxation, attach a temperature-sensing device to your fingers; try to raise the temperature as you induce relaxation. Or attach a GSR device to a comfortable part of the body, and work to lower your skin conductivity as you relax. You can use a heart-rate counter in the same way. "Try" and "work at" are actually misleading—what's involved in biofeedback is less a matter of will than of more or less *intending* to lower hand temperature of whatever, and letting it happen. The important thing is that the device will tell you when you're successfully relaxing, offering concrete signs of progress. Try your imaging exercises while in a state of deep relaxation aided by biofeedback. If necessary, open your eyes briefly, or have readings read to you in a soft voice.

You may also want to try biofeedback to deepen the benefits of the ideal imaginary environment. Was coolness or warmth a part of the environment? If your hands feel best when warm, for example, use biofeedback to find when you're warming them most effectively (the same thing works if you're trying to imagine a cooling environment). It's easiest to use this kind of equipment on the hands, feet, arms, and legs, but you can attach the temperature sensor to your trunk or head if that's the area that needs relief. The changes in temperature won't be as striking on central parts of your body as on the extremities. But remember the Houseplant Effect and the big difference a small change can make.

One thing to keep firmly in mind: biofeedback is only a tool. *You* are achieving the results that the device is merely measuring. It's just one more way of tapping your ability to take control of your own body. If you get nothing more from biofeedback than a graphic demonstration that you can raise or lower your hand temperature or relax the surface of your skin, you've gotten a great deal. Now go back to your relaxation and imaging exercises with the confidence that you deserve.

16

Psychotherapy: Help in Depth

Like hypnosis, psychotherapy has had image problems. It's not Svengali this time, but a bearded gentleman who occasionally murmurs "Aha!" as his supine patient prattles aimlessly or a California smoothie who exhorts his followers to exorcise all their frustrations in a single scream. Some people fear that therapy, like hypnosis, means surrendering one's will and becoming dependent, or they consider it an extreme step, something only for the certifiably off-the-wall.

These misgivings and misconceptions are unfortunate, because they keep many people from a powerful resource for improving their lives. I'm biased, of course, because psychotherapy is my work, but I never cease to be amazed at the good it can do for a host of emotional difficulties as well as skin problems. If it were not for my own psychotherapy at a young age, I doubt very much that I'd be in any position to help others—or write books.

Will psychotherapy—with a psychologist, psychiatrist, or social worker—help your skin? Like hypnosis, psychotherapy sounds mysterious but has a lot in common with events and experiences of daily life: conversations with compassionate friends and neighbors (even a supportive bartender or hairdresser) who help you put your problems in perspective; solitary afternoons in a basement workshop or on a mountain trail.

The essence of psychotherapy is *looking inward*. It's an intellectual and emotional process (I'd say about 15 percent the former, 85 percent the latter) that helps connect your feelings and your life. It aims to help you feel *more* of your feelings. As I said earlier, the emotions you *don't* feel—your longing for love, your urgent need for protection, your anger—are often a main ingredient in skin problems; they are triggers, hooks that keep them holding on, magnifiers that intensify their impact.

You already know a good bit about psychotherapy if you've been doing the diagnostic exercises of Part I. Getting to know the advantages of your symptom and the emotional tasks it performs, imagining "What if it got worse?" and putting your illness into the context of the rest of your life on a Time Line—you're looking inward to the needs, wishes, and fears that have become entangled with the condition of your skin.

Insight is its own reward—it's fascinating to know yourself better, and finding links between separate parts of your life is like solving an immensely challenging mystery novel. But self-knowledge is only the first step. To change through psychotherapy, you must *feel* the emotions you've thought you had to push aside. And this requires courage and perseverance. The feelings you buried were painful, or else you'd never have buried them. It's like trying to solve a mystery while you secretly fear that the criminal will prove to be yourself.

When therapy works, however, a lot more than pain is involved. The same courage that lets us feel more of our pain allows us to feel more of the joy of life. Increasing our ability to feel more of the pleasure, warmth, and fullness of life is as much a goal as reducing the pain.

Sometimes, insight and change occur dramatically. A man may be screaming furiously at his wife—a repeated scenario of their marriage—when she tells him: "Right now, you sound exactly like your father. I can imagine how you used to feel when *he* screamed at *you*." Struck by her perception, he doesn't simply see the resemblance, he *feels* it: he remembers the pain, fear, and frustrated fury he buried as a small boy at the receiving end of his father's anger. He experiences yesterday's pain in today's outburst. He can still scream at his wife, but never again with that same tormented fury: knowing where feelings come from robs them of despotic power and puts you in a position to change how you act as well as feel.

Such sudden flashes of insight are the exception, and usually come only after a period of behind-the-scenes preparation. This man had been preoccupied with the problems posed by his anger for some time and was ready to see the truth when it was presented to him. He had found the courage to once again be the little boy terrified by his father's temper, and this relieved him of the need to repeatedly "rewrite history" by taking the role of his angry father. He can now begin the adventure of really knowing his wife, unshackled from history.

A similar process may help you free yourself from the grip of your symptom. Recognizing how the emotional task of "seeking love and affection" is involved in your allergies, for example, may foster a quest to understand its roots in a childhood that didn't provide the love you needed. From insight comes the courage to experience directly those childhood emotions that express themselves in adult problems.

It's not a matter of rewriting your history—no one can do that—but changing your relationship to it, allowing it to fall back into the past. Dr. Alfred Adler, a great pioneer of psychiatry, called the process of psychotherapy "spitting in the soup of neurosis: you can still drink it, but it never tastes the same." Once you've experienced the painful emotions that generate today's rash, uncontrollable temper, or series of doomed relationships, you can continue to live the same way, but you no longer *have* to. Your past has lost its old power over you.

Change is part of life, and we often achieve liberating insight spontaneously as we grow and mature. Supportive friends who care about you can be helpful, but a professional psychotherapist is *trained* to help you get there. To know that you're not alone in your struggle—that someone understands and appreciates what you're going through—lightens any burden. A good therapist will be a constant reminder that there's nothing weird, exaggerated, or unnecessary about your reaction to your symptom: you're dealing with old as well as new problems. When you're working with a therapist, you needn't worry about being self-absorbed or a burden, which is natural when your troubles dominate conversations with friends. In fact, many say that therapy improves friendships by taking some of the heat off them.

A therapist can be supportive in a special way. Change requires giving up safe, tested ways of living and trying to do things differently, while somewhere within you remains the fear of the child you were: if you get angry, retribution will follow; if you feel your sexuality, everyone around you will be appalled and accusatory. In therapy you have a safe testing ground where you can try out your emerging self with a trustworthy support at your side, and see for yourself that nothing unthinkable actually happens. It is common, for example, for a patient to express anger at a therapist; this doesn't mean therapy has failed, but that it is working. It is providing a precious opportunity to test the experience of anger—to feel it, to gain insight into where it comes from, to see that no dreadful retribution follows.

But does psychotherapy actually work for skin problems? This is not a simple question, and research in the field is inconsistent. Some psychotherapists consider skin patients poor candidates for therapy, but case histories and controlled experiments have documented substantial benefits for many people. Perhaps the only reasonable answer is: sometimes, for some people. Just like medicine. Let's look at some of the research results to help you gauge if it may help you.

At the University Medical Center in Indianapolis, for example, twenty-five patients with various skin irritations, including dermatitis and neurotic excoriation, were given short-term psychotherapy in twelve weekly sessions. Therapy is usually tailored to the individual patient, but this focused on issues the doctors expected to be most relevant: unexpressed rage and unexpressed wishes for love.

During the twelve sessions, doctors encouraged patients to put their anger into words, without guilt; to see links between their early lives and their current relationships; to deal more directly with their feelings.

The results were striking. As angry feelings came to the surface, patients felt understandably more upset—and their skin often got briefly worse. Then, as they learned to express these angry feelings directly, their skin began to improve. Among the thirteen patients who stuck with the therapy program all the way through, twelve enjoyed substantial gains in their skin problem—gains that remained long after the experiment was over.

In this sense, the experiment was a success. On the other hand, the dropout rate was extremely high: nearly half the patients didn't make it through the program.[1] This underscores an essential point: to be effective, therapy must be tailored to the individual. The short-term, intense, and demanding therapy used here simply wasn't right for half the participants. *They* were right in leaving. They might have done better with a slower, less intensive type of therapy. Or it could be that they weren't ready for therapy at that time; they were not yet able to look at their anger and their needs directly enough to make changes.

That therapy works only for those who need and are ready for it was implied by another study, this one from England. Here, one group of eczema patients was given the standard dermatological treatment; another group, dermatology plus up to four months of psychotherapy.

This therapy was more individualized. It aimed to help patients deal with conflicts and frustrations, and make them more aware of their hostility and other disturbing emotions.

Results were not dramatically impressive overall. The psychotherapy group experienced only slightly greater skin improvements than the control group. But a look at individual participants was far more encouraging. Those people who had had psychological or physical symptoms before their eczema developed—who apparently had some prior emotional problems— got better *twice* as fast as controls. *And they were the ones who hadn't improved at all with earlier dermatological treatment alone.*[2]

This study suggests a simple conclusion: if there is an emotional dimension to your skin problem, psychotherapy is essential; if not, it will have little impact. However, don't overlook the fact that any skin problem, even if its origins are more physical, will cause its own emotional turmoil, and many sufferers will gain substantially from the support of a knowledgeable, sympathetic therapist, though they will most likely feel the gains in their hearts, not their skins.

The support function of therapy was clear in a study at the

University of Pennsylvania, in which ten patients with severe, recurrent oral herpes—cold sores—were given a series of psychoanalytically oriented therapy sessions. For all these patients, physical treatments of all sorts had proved ineffective, and it had been established that specific emotional events could trigger outbreaks.

Improvement in the severity of the symptom and in the patients' state of mind was noted as early as the second session. Clearly, no major personality change or profound insight had taken place. What was involved here was probably just the presence of a caring, concerned, reassuring individual. Several patients, in fact, suffered recurrences when the therapist was unexpectedly absent.[3]

The importance of the *relationship* with the therapist reflects the fact that relationships are central in many skin problems—I think of them as diseases of two or more people, although only one has the symptoms. Often the disorder involves mother and child first, and is later duplicated in marriage.

Many skin problems improve with therapy or counseling that focuses on relationships rather than individuals. In one clinical study, a group of fifty-three children with chronic eczema received medical care plus mother-and-child counseling in which a psychologist explained how the child's emotional needs could best be met. A control group received medical care alone. The children who had counseling did significantly better than those who did not.[4]

Whether you've been getting good or not-so-good results with this book, you might want to consider working with a psychotherapist. Many people find the process of insight and change goes more quickly with the aid of a trained professional. Even if you're ready to do the work yourself, a therapist can help you as a coach helps an athlete, with encouragement and advice on your technique and timing.

Don't be deterred by the mistaken notion that therapy is only for weak individuals who can't make it through life on their own. Virtually anyone can, at some point, gain from the professional help a good therapist can offer. And don't let the profusion of therapies that have developed in recent decades overwhelm you with the tasks of choosing the one that's just right for you. Studies have found that experienced therapists, whatever their original training, actually do pretty much the same things in therapy. If you feel ready for this kind of assistance, you'll find practical suggestions of getting it in Appendix II.

17

Breaking the Itch-Scratch Cycle

I was handcuffed, chained, or tied to my bed at night to try to prevent me from scratching. I was even put in a straitjacket to stop me from ripping the ever present bandages off and opening up the wounds which never got a chance to heal. But Harry Houdini was my hero. I always escaped any bondage and clawed myself to a bloody mess before I fell asleep, exhausted. They kept telling me I'd have scars, but I didn't care. I couldn't control myself. I always had dark circles under my eyes, I never got enough sleep. I was always missing school, and even when I went, I often had to be sent home because I'd made a bloody mess of myself again, picking off the scabs under the bandage.

I literally had no friends outside my family. I hardly ever left the house. Everyone was afraid to touch me.

My condition was very severe from soon after birth to about age fourteen. I was taken to practically every doctor and quack in the area. I was in and out of hospitals every year. My family spent thousands of dollars on treatment that never afforded more than temporary relief.

My strongest memories are of crying myself to sleep every night. My mother would come in and rock me and reassure me that she loved me and that maybe tomorrow there would be a miracle and I would be all better. I prayed for that miracle and waited for that miracle for a long time. Then I just stopped believing in God.[1]

This young woman's description of the itching that twisted and constricted her childhood sounds extreme. But anyone who has been caught in the itch-scratch cycle will recognize her torment.

It can have many causes. This woman's diagnosis was atopic dermatitis—eczema. Some medical illnesses produce itching: diabetes, liver disease, kidney problems, or reactions to medications. So do simple insect bites. Itching can accompany eruptions of eczema, psoriasis, and hives or torment skin that looks perfectly healthy.[2]

Is your itch medical or psychological? You and your doctors could pursue this fruitless question for years, and you'll be itching all the while. So get the best medical work-up and treatment you can, but remember: *all itching is ultimately psychological*. However intense, regardless of origin, itching is not a disease but an experience: it has no physical reality that even the most diligent of scientists can find. Using negative hypnosis techniques, researchers have produced itching in a healthy arm that had been fully anesthetized—that was unable to *physically* feel anything.

This is certainly not to dismiss itching as "all in your head." It's every bit as real as pain; the most agonizing pain has no detectable physical form, either, but no one argues that all pain is imaginary. Significantly, the sensation of itching is carried by the same nerve fibers that carry pain.[3] Both pain and itching may have physical causes, whose impact is aggravated by psychological factors.

If you find it hard to believe that emotions can make you itch, consider the most prosaic itch in the world: a mosquito bite. You get this particular bite toward the end of a glorious day at the beach. You're enjoying witty conversation with old friends on the drive home, and looking forward to a good dinner. The bite itches, but your attention is quickly distracted by the pleasures of the moment. The physical reality of the bite has virtually no impact.

Suppose the next Sunday at the beach isn't so glorious. The crowds come early, the overcast stays late, radios are blaring, and someone forgot the beer. It's still hot and humid as you drive back to the city, where your air conditioner is still broken, thanks to that rotten landlord. But this is something you won't have to worry about for a while, because the traffic is stalled. Your companions make the Mickey Mouse Club sound like the Academy of Science.

You have another mosquito bite. But this time, without pleasant distractions your attention focuses on it like a searchlight. All the frustration of the day fuels your irritation. The more you itch the more you scratch and the more you scratch the more you itch. As the blood starts to ooze you know you are caught in the cycle.

If frustration, anger, and anxiety can magnify the itch of a simple mosquito bite, you can imagine what emotions can do to the itch of eczema or psoriasis. When the searchlight of consciousness fastens on an area of the skin, it becomes the scapegoat for a lifetime of insults. The results can be devastating.

The question uppermost in the mind of most itch sufferers is a simple one: "How can I make it go away?" As with pain, while medical treatments often help, the big surprise is the effectiveness of psychological techniques. Hypnosis and similar pain-control methods have proved effective enough for some people to go through major surgery with no medication at all. The same power can be used to tame an itch.

The first step in treating any itch should be a good medical evaluation. Your dermatologist or allergist may discover "trigger factors" in your diet and environment, and encourage you to minimize or eliminate them. He may suggest wearing different clothes or washing them in a different detergent, and avoiding certain foods and chemicals. If there is an underlying disease like diabetes, he will refer you to a specialist for treatment.

Beyond that, medical care simply aims to reduce the itch itself. Anti-itch baths and tar ointments suppress inflammation and lubricate the skin; antihistamines such as Atarax relieve some itching by breaking the biochemical chain. Most frequently used nowadays are the corticosteroids, such as cortisone, which reduce the inflammation that intensifies itching. (Mild forms of these creams are now available over the counter.)[4] For many people, these conventional approaches are not enough.

The psychological techniques in this book will relieve itching regardless of cause—even when it's as medical as liver disease. In fact, it appears that itching with a clear and specific medical cause responds best to psychological intervention, because there is less emotional reluctance to "let go."[5]

The psychological and medical approaches work well together. Relaxation, for example, can help you to get more relief out of less cortisone, letting you avoid the feeling of dependence many people get as their steroid cream takes a central role in their lives.

Psychological itch control has four parts: (1) Breaking the skin code to understand and respond to the medical and/or psychological message that your body is screaming with its symptom. (2) Relaxation to relieve the tensions that aggravate the itch. (3) Life changes to alleviate situational stresses. (4) Breaking the itch-scratch cycle.

Itching can reflect any of the eleven tasks listed in Chapter 2. The dictionary definition of itching, "a constant irritating desire or longing," is often right on target. I've often found that itchy skin is hard at work on the task of "looking for love and protection." A "maddening itch" is another accurate figure of speech that hints at anger beneath the surface. Is your skin taking a beating? Metaphorically, we are "feeling itchy" when we are no longer content but not yet ready to act. Many a literal itch strikes people caught in this life bind.

The basic emotional push behind itching and scratching is always a healthy one. The scratching, picking, or tearing is an attempt at self-help, directed at one of the tasks or at the skin itself. We scratch to reduce the itch. The intent is honorable but the technique is terrible. Similarly, the picking and tearing so typical of people with acne is an attempt to improve the skin. The intent is fine, the technique ineffective.

We also talk of sexual frustration as "feeling itchy." Itching—particularly in the genital and anal areas—frequently means the skin is working on the task of seeking love or dealing with more complicated sexual conflicts. The logic can be startlingly clear.

Tim, a thirty-five-year-old consultant, suffered a kind of ultra jock itch that took the form of a red, burning ring from his anus to the top of his penis. Looser underwear, a milder laundry soap, and cortisone cream helped. But no dermatologist had managed to find a medical cause, and nothing had made it go away.

Through persistently listening to his skin and observing his Time Line, Tim finally gained insight into the symptom's hidden meaning. The itch appeared whenever a setback undermined his sense of potency. An unsolvable problem at work might start the fire. It worsened when his wife undercut him in conversation and flared up when she refused his sexual overtures. "Every time I feel that someone is trying to cut my balls off, I get the burning ring. It's as if they'd actually done it," Tim realized. His insight marked the beginning of steady, substantial improvement. Working mostly on his own, he achieved 90 percent relief of symptoms. When a major life crisis triggered a major recurrence, he overcame it with psychological techniques. Now, whenever the itch begins to smolder, he quenches it with some self-therapy and a bit of mild steroid cream.

As Tim struggled with an itch that he didn't scratch, some people scratch without itching. There may have once been an itch that started the cycle, but the scratching has long continued on its own momentum.

For Donna, a forty-year-old mother of four teenagers, the problem *seemed* to be small, relentlessly itching bumps on her legs, buttocks, stomach, and arms. Twelve years of dermatology, creams, lotions, baths, and pills had occasionally helped, but never resolved the problem. She was frustrated, angry, and disappointed with herself and her doctors. And she was still tearing at her skin.

It was a consulting dermatologist, Dr. Kenneth Arndt of Boston's Beth Israel Hospital, who suggested that the problem lay less in Donna's bumps than in her reaction to them. "She has no primary disease of the skin, but a difficult habit pattern," he pointed out. The bumps would be a mild condition were she not constantly tearing and squeezing them.

The search for medical diagnosis and medication to eliminate the bumps gave way to a quest for the emotional cause of Donna's scratching, and psychological techniques to control it. We quickly identified a key source of irritation in Donna's life: her husband. He was distant, withdrawn, and sexually demanding—a combination that left her feeling used. She was caught between her anger and her inability to confront him. After several sessions, Donna came to see how her skin had been waving a red flag to express the frustrated feelings she couldn't feel directly: it was ceaselessly itching to change. Her "itchy" feelings started to

move from her skin to a mix of anxiety, anger, and sexual excitement as she began to take a more direct, even combative approach with her husband.

But Donna needed more immediate help. She learned to
practice a relaxation exercise, and spent less time scratching. She
developed her ideal imaginary environment: a cool, soothing
swimming pool. Effective as these techniques were, she needed
still more help. Any time she succumbed to the impulse to scratch,
it started an avalanche. Her scratching became frenzied, and she
became terrified she'd lost all her new gains. So Donna and I developed two other techniques that finally helped break her twelve-
year habit. I'd like to teach them to you.

(A word of warning: these advanced techniques won't give
maximum relief if you haven't learned the diagnostic and treatment exercises of earlier chapters. You still need to work through
the emotional and life issues that fuel your problem; you need to
enter the healing state regularly, luxuriating in your ideal imaginary environement.)

UNLINKING THE CHAIN

Itches are like chains: shake any link and every link rattles. Scratch
your wrist and soon a cascade of itching will pour down your
arm, over your shoulder, and across your chest. This sets up a
black-and-white situation: either your mastery is perfect, or you
slip irreversibly into total itching. You need the freedom to itch
or scratch *a bit* without falling back to zero.

1. Do your usual sequence, relax, enter the healing state, and
   sample the soothing pleasure of the ideal imaginary environment.
2. Loosely focus on the image of a length of chain. But imagine
   that each link of this chain is totally separate from the others.
   No matter how vigorously you shake it, one link can't budge
   any other link.

This image helps your mind and body unlearn the expectation that the first itch or scratch unleashes the whole cycle.

Don't work or push at this image. Plant it like a seed each
time you do the series of exercises. "Water" the seed a hundred

times a day by letting yourself see the image of an unlinked chain for a fraction of a second. Take some of the energy that you throw into your typical inner monologue of doubt and fear and use it instead to fertilize the seed, the image.

You can put this image to work in many ways:

1. Unlink the itch on the side of your knee from the skin on the front and back of your knee and all over your body. Even if you were to scratch the side of your knee a bit, it wouldn't matter. The experience is totally separate from all other itches and scratches.

2. Unlink *today's* itch or scratch from all your yesterdays. Imagine that each itch means no more to you than the most incidental itch would mean to someone who had never heard of the itch-scratch cycle. Unlink it from the difficult time in your life when the problem started. Separate *now* from history.

3. Unlink the *urge* to scratch from the action: let it simply remain an urge. If you can observe, "Ah yes, there's that old urge, ho hum," you have disconnected it from any action or emotion.

4. Unlink the rest of yourself from the itchy piece of skin. Imagine it floating across the room. It has nothing to do with you.

5. Step outside of yourself. See the person over there who is struggling with an itch. Observe that he or she looks exactly like you. Wish him or her good luck. Then move on to something else.

6. Most important of all: unlink your skin from its assigned task. Let your head and heart do the longing; express the anger; feel the sexual feelings. Let your skin be skin.

Now stop. Let yourself benefit from the unlinked-chain techniques for at least a few days before going on.

SCRATCHING HAND TO SOOTHING HAND

You've been trying to stop scratching with willpower? It simply won't work. Your itch keeps building, keeps calling out for help. Your hand finally reaches to relieve it, almost of its own accord. The hand is quicker than the will.

Why can't you just tell yourself to stop scratching? Very simple: *you* never told yourself to start. Your conscious willpower self isn't running the show.

Then who is in charge here? Neither your conscious mind nor your unconscious mind. You don't direct the scratching, but you're not unaware of it either. Your scratch control center is directly linked to the healing part of the mind that we've been exploring throughout the book. But as you well know by now, if you want help from this part of yourself, you have to speak its language. You can't push, work, or insist. You need to be subtle and wily.

For example, try to *not* think of a hippopotamus. Now try harder. Bulldozing yourself with willpower is not effective. Now have each hippopotamus turn into an elephant. Much easier?

Rather than struggling to restrain your scratching hand, you can convert it: you can turn the pesky hippopotamus into a loyal, powerful elephant of an ally.

At the very moment your hand reaches to scratch, it is transformed into a soothing embodiment of your ideal imaginary environment. You can learn to do this conversion as automatically as you once learned to catch a ball: you don't do it—your hand itself does. You can use this technique as you would use steroid cream, to gain control over your itch. Once you break the cycle, you may find that your skin heals itself.

It probably took you years to learn to catch a ball smoothly and without thinking. But you can learn to transform your scratching hand into a healing hand through daily practice sessions with the help of the healing state.

1. Using your own customized method, relax and induce the healing state.
2. Experience your ideal imaginary environment.
3. Unlink the chain.
4. Imagine your hand as a deep reservoir of whatever sensations are most healing and soothing for your skin. When your hand is full almost to the bursting point, move it to each of the areas that sometimes itch. Just rest the soothing hand lightly on your skin. You needn't rub or press. Feel the soothing sensations flow out your fingers, taking over so totally that there is no room at all for an itch. Give each area as much help as it needs.

If your hand needs replenishing, just take it away from your skin and let it fill up again. You can repeat the procedure as often as needed.

5. Focus on the idea that your scratching hand will be *automatically* transformed into a soothing hand. In the middle of its flight, before hitting the target, your hand will become a healing instrument.

Go through the procedure at least daily, preferably twice a day. *Be prepared for a discouraging period before you master this challenging but ultimately effortless mental magic.* When it works—when your hand reaches for an itch and automatically soothes with a touch—you'll feel more like an amazed spectator than someone who's "broken a habit" by heroic willpower.

You can't work at these techniques any more than you can convince a flower to grow faster by cheering it on. Plant the seed of each technique, feed it with relaxation and repetition. (If it starts to feel more like work than a personal gift to yourself, take a day off.) To add momentum to the learning process, take a fraction of a second a hundred times a day to remind yourself, "unlinked chain" and "scratching hand to soothing hand."

Nighttime itching is a particular torment.[6] A good night's sleep becomes a distant memory, as mind and body ache for rest. Why is scratching such a problem at night? I suspect it's the absence of daytime distractions. At night we are back to basics, our wishes and fears, our bed partners, our body's aches and itches.

In the past, you've continued scratching all through the night, even though your conscious mind was asleep. In the same way, the soothing hand technique will keep on working now. The scratching hand used to awaken you, but the soothing hand will protect your sleep and dreams. Because you're only a spectator, the conversion will go on whether you are asleep or awake.

What's true of most skin disorders is rarely clearer than with itching: you're an active part of the problem and you must participate in the solution. There is real magic in these techniques. But even a master magician has to practice. That demands energy, but much less energy than you've been putting into itching and scratching.

PART THREE

Is It
Working?

18

Holding On/Letting Go: Your Symptom's Last Stand

By now you've read thousands of words to help you understand your skin problem and worked hard on exercises to release yourself from its grip. The big question in your mind is no doubt a practical one: *Is it working?* Particularly if earlier efforts to get well have left a long chain of disappointments, or you still suspect that there's something flaky in a psychological approach to what you've always been told is a physical problem.

"Is it working?" is a delicate question with this kind of therapy. My mind-body approach isn't designed to get the quick, dramatic results that can follow a shot of steroids or an antibiotic. Signs of progress can take many forms, including some that easily escape your notice.

It's a critical question because stalls and slowdowns in progress are very common in this kind of therapy. Psychotherapists call it *resistance*, and it means your symptom is *holding on* despite your efforts. It's not a sign of failure, but a great opportunity to understand the needs, fears, and emotional tasks that give the symptom its power. Just to recognize that you're holding on can be a major breakthrough.

"Is it working?" can be hard to answer because individual responses to therapy vary so widely. I've found that most skin patients get at least some results in six to twelve weekly sessions. But the range is enormous. One patient who had a rash around his genitals worked (mainly on his own) through four years of improvements and plateaus before he reached the point where he was symptom-free 90 percent of the time; another reported her warts disappeared immediately after she called me for an appointment!

What expectations are realistic? As a general rule (exceptions are numerous), the longer you've had the problem, the longer it will take to leave. Jean, whose eczema dates from birth, may get as good results as Jane, whose skin was fine until last February, but it will probably take a lot more time and energy to get there. Similarly, a severe, widespread rash will probably demand more effort than a limited eruption.

Symptoms on the central body—chest, stomach, back, or genitals—seem to take the longest to get better. Those on the head and neck are more tractable, and those on the hands and feet respond quickest of all. Perhaps the subtle physiological changes of relaxation and hypnosis are most readily achieved in areas farthest from the body's center. Or the body symbolism we discussed in Chapter 7 plays a part: it takes more work to dislodge symptoms closest to the heart, head, and gut.

You are another critical factor. Younger people are usually in a more active state of flux and formation than their elders, and this gives them a head start in making changes. When skin symptoms are tied to a time of upheaval—adolescence, divorce—they often improve quickly. If your symptom is a persistent annoyance in an otherwise satisfactory settled existence, gains will probably come more slowly than they will to a person whose whole life is distressed and in turmoil—who feels he's absolutely *had it* with his symptom and must make something happen.

I get the impression that patients do best who've had particularly *poor* results with conventional dermatology and are ready to embrace something completely different. If you still believe that some wonder pill might come out of a laboratory tomorrow or that Dr. Right is in the next professional building, you're likely to be more tentative with the work we're doing here.

Remember that progress can take many shapes and forms. The disease itself may improve in one way or another: the rash disappears or attacks are shorter and less frequent; you continue to have flare-ups but in smaller areas. Your symptom may be unchanged but you *suffer* less: itching, burning, or pain are not the torment they once were; they no longer rule your life. Or it may be emotional impact that's reduced: less shame, fear, revulsion, or sense that your life and body are out of your control. This intangible improvement is progress just as sure and significant as a drop in the number of pustules.

If you're discouraged and uncertain whether my approach is working at all, make sure your eyes are open to changes on all three fronts. I'd recommend going through all the diagnostic material and then using treatment exercises for at least three weeks—with lots of energy and commitment—before making any judgment. If *absolutely* nothing has happened, it could be this kind of treatment has nothing to offer you. (In my experience, this is extremely rare.) Check your condition, using the Micro Time Line and the Griesemer scale of Chapter 5, and review the Introduction and Time Line exercises (Chapter 5) for any indication that your symptom may be emotionally responsive.

Only if the results are uniformly negative—no progress of any sort, no suggestion that your skin has any link to your head and heart, a low percentage on the Griesemer scale—would I start to think that you have nothing to gain from my program. Otherwise, before passing this book onto another afflicted friend or a tag sale, I'd give serious thought to the possibility that you're *holding on*.

What's happening, in this case, is that the same power that has kept your symptom entrenched for months or years is now redoubling its efforts against your attempts to dislodge it. There's no weakness or blame here. Consciously, you want to be well, but the wishes, fears, and needs under the skin are intent on roadblocks and sabotage. A certain amount of holding on is inevitable when treatment efforts come close to home. Rather than flagellate yourself, have some respect for the strength of your inner self.

A colleague, Dr. Richard Pomerance, compares holding on to the Japanese soldier who appears as a stock character in old movies. Detached from his unit during jungle fighting in the Pacific, he's taken refuge in a cave. He's sworn to defend the emperor and empire to the death, and his commander once warned him that one day people might tempt him to surrender with false reports that the emperor was dead and the war lost. He must never listen to them! Sure enough, he continues to hole up in his cave, years after the war is over. Villagers try to convince him that his struggle has lost all meaning, but he can't forget his oath; he remains convinced that these reports are just enemy propaganda.

Many symptoms are like the soldier in the story. They were once enlisted to defend the vulnerable ego against the pain of unmet needs, fears, and troubling emotions. The war is now over and the symptom serves no one by keeping up its lonely fight. But it will not be convinced: its devotion to a cause of the past is unshakable. All our attempts to make it let go—the gamut of treatments here—are like the reports that the soldier disbelieves. The symptom continually throws up roadblocks to protect its "emperor" by making sure that no therapy works.

Such roadblocks can be quite concrete. Judy D., a teacher, came to me with painful plantar warts on her right foot. She'd been through such therapies as freezing and acid, but nothing worked for long. We got off to a fine start with hypnosis; the first night she tried self-hypnosis, she said, she saw that it might have a major impact.

But from that point onward, things got difficult. She missed appointments, blaming heavy traffic en route to the office. She arrived for one session with her arm so painfully strained from softball the day before that she couldn't raise it above her shoulder—and thus could not practice the arm levitation that was part of her hypnotic procedure. Judy insisted she was eager to continue with therapy, but her actions said something different.

As we discussed the history of her warts one day, an important clue emerged. The first doctor who treated them was the father of a friend, who used an effective but extremely painful therapy. Shortly afterward, the doctor died. In adulthood, the warts came out of remission following the death of a colleague.

My guess was that the child Judy had been very angry with her first doctor for the pain he caused—a natural reaction—and then felt secretly responsible and guilty when he died. The later death of her colleague rekindled the feeling. When it became clear that my treatment might make the warts go away, she panicked:

the last time that happened, someone died! She'd never dealt directly with the painful feelings of that childhood episode, or with earlier guilts and fears that were tied in with it. Holding on to the warts was less painful than confronting the feelings that had overwhelmed her as a child and in the timeless parts of her heart and mind overwhelmed her still.

Often, holding on serves the same emotional task that gives the symptom its power. Joseph K., a thirty-year-old teacher, had atopic eczema from infancy through early childhood, then hay fever until his teens, when eczema took over again. Outwardly, Joseph was a most compliant patient, but however hard he tried to please, no therapy ever worked for long. When he worked with me it became clear that despite his best intentions, he could follow his exercise program only in fits and starts.

I saw that this pattern had a special meaning in Joseph's life. His mother had been an extremely controlling woman, and he'd always passively complied with her demands, despite a boiling anger that never reached the surface. With his wife, his neighbors, his kids, he was relentlessly Mr. Nice Guy, agreeable on the surface and eager to please—although his natural drive for adult independence had never withered away.

In therapy he was similarly all cooperation up front. Yet with me, as with a series of dermatologists, he harbored the same underground resistance that had protected his autonomy against his mother, and then his wife. Giving up the symptom because of *my* efforts would be, in a sense, giving up his soul.

An important turning point came when I suggested to Joseph that his scratching was the healthiest part of his life. His mother told him to stop; his wife told him to stop; first his dermatologist and now his psychotherapist tried to make him stop. But he kept on scratching! This was one place where he was his own man.

Pointing out to Joseph K. that scratching was indeed an act of vigorous independence ironically enabled him to stop. Around the same time, he reported that turmoil was coming to the surface in his relationship with his wife. In a surprising display of autonomy, he announced that he wanted to continue work on his skin alone—using the techniques we'd developed in therapy—and the last I heard he was doing well.

Recognizing your own holding on may open the door to self-knowledge: if you can come to grips with the feelings you're protecting yourself from, you'll give your efforts a major boost. Exploring the roots of holding on can yield the same inner information as the dreams, daydreams, and other diagnostic exercises of Part I.

Holding on often feels as if it's *happening* to you—you just can't find the time for the exercises, you're interrupted, or something is preventing you from concentrating. A critical first step is acknowledging that you yourself are doing it—on some level, that is, you are *actively* holding on.

How can you clue yourself into the process?

The first question is simple. Are you really doing the work? Have you done both diagnostic and treatment exercises seriously, consistently, in an atmosphere free from interruption? Or did you give them a quick once-over, then shelve them for later? Did you run through them superficially and conclude that nothing would happen? Did you always seem to be interrupted? What seems like force of circumstance—"I just can't find the time or place"—is often holding on.

Frequently, people report that they give the exercises their best shot but nothing happens. "Nothing comes to my mind. It's a blank," they say. The mind constantly produces thoughts, feelings, images, and associations—to make it truly blank is a capacity that yogis and mystics spend years developing. So ask yourself: "What is *creating* this blank in my mind? What feelings or thoughts am I avoiding? What pain am I backing off from?" Let your mind drift over the notion "I'm avoiding something," and see what occurs to you.

You may feel that you've been an exemplary patient. You do the diagnostic exercises conscientiously, and as you do, all sorts of painful, fascinating, guilty revelations bubble up. Yet you don't *feel* that anything's happening. This may be because you're not feeling the emotions that belong to the memories: your exercises are all head and no heart. Despite the magnitude of your surface efforts and effects, inside you're backing away—or holding on. You're like a person who's afraid of heights but who forces himself to climb mountains—he's done something difficult, but he's still afraid of heights at the end of the day! People who hold on in this way were often good little boys and girls, straight-A students, and model workers—despite the troubles and dissents boiling within.

Because holding on—resistance—is so widespread in psychotherapy, it has been extensively studied, and we can use some of these insights. Dr. Ralph Greenson has compiled the classic signs that holding on is taking place.[1] Among them:

• Either you experience no emotion as important information emerges (see above) or the emotions are inappropriate: you giggle when you think of something sad, or your eyes water when you remember something happy.

• Postures are a clue. As you work on the exercises, you hunch into a stiff, rigid posture; your fists clench, your neck muscles tighten, your feet curl up. Or you perform repetitive movements: your feet bounce, your head nods, your fingers tap.

• You often find yourself drowsing and falling asleep during the exercises.

• There are conspicuous gaps and omissions. You dredge up lots of memories about your father and sisters, but nothing about your mother, or a particular brother. Nothing that relates to anger, or to sexuality, ever seems to come up.

• You approach diagnostic or therapeutic exercises rigidly, concentrating on them at a particular time of day, but forgetting them utterly otherwise. It's as if you're encapsulating the effort to keep it from permeating your entire life. (If you're not holding on this way, it's almost inevitable that passing thoughts about therapy will occur to you throughout the day.)

• One or more avenues of insight seem closed to you. That is, you're picking up diagnostic clues from your daydreams, family photographs, and the like, but you can never remember early life events.

• Cheerfulness and enthusiasm, though usually praiseworthy and pleasant, may indicate holding on. If you find yourself telling everyone of the terrific book you're reading and the exciting discoveries you're making about yourself, take a step back and consider: a lot of what I'm asking you to do is demanding and painful. Why hasn't it dampened your enthusiasm—at least a little bit?

Your style of holding on may point to the emotional needs or fears at the bottom of it. Are you constantly peeking ahead, reading bits and pieces of various chapters before getting down to work? Skimming is fair enough, unless you do it *instead* of getting down to work. You might ask yourself if you're generally prone to the superficial once-over: do you avoid the full force of suspense by checking out the end of mystery novels before it gets too intense? You may be avoiding full emotional commitment in the same way here.

Or perhaps you're not following the program in proper sequence because you're struggling for control; the adolescent within you is digging in his heels in reaction to the idea that "somebody's telling me what to do." Consider going through the book in an orderly, methodical manner. Does the image bother you?

Some people start off great guns and then peter out. After four days of serious, sustained diagnostic work, they no longer can find time to continue, until they finally lose all momentum. Have you seen this pattern elsewhere in your life? Does a siege of self-doubt often torpedo promising progress?

It could be that initial gains are checked by a fear of success: it may be threatening to think of yourself as an effective heavyweight rather than a dilettante. Remaining an incompetent child is a way of protecting yourself from the anger of adults or the retribution of a wrathful parent who exists only in the timeless mind.

Others report a similar pattern in which a little progress ends in a plateau, or even a backslide: it feels impossible to secure temporary gains. It may be that progress ends when the emotional ante gets too high; that's when the lone soldier barricades himself within his cave. Try to come to terms with whatever it is within that limits your ability to change and confront emotions. Did you taper off when results were too good? Or did you find yourself growing fearful and anxious as results began to show? What fears were stirred up within you? What boat was rocked?

Some of my patients first report frustration: "I'm working— but the techniques aren't." They've put serious, consistent effort into both diagnostic and therapeutic exercises, they've engaged their hearts as well as their minds in the effort—but the impact has been zero.

My advice for these people is to look systematically and objectively at the three areas in which change takes place: the physical symptom, your subjective experience of it, and its emotional impact. Ask friends and family if they've noted any change for the better—any change at all in you or your skin. Do you seem more relaxed, more cheerful, easier to live with? Being blind to improvements often means holding on to your sense of yourself as sick.

If your feeling that the book has failed is accompanied by acute disappointment, ask yourself if this seems familiar. Do you often feel you're being set up, promised the moon and then let down? Am I just the latest in a series of unclothed emperors? If so, you might wonder if all these are echoes of childhood, when a supremely important emperor left you in the lurch when you needed him or her. People can become so used to their rhythm of great expectations and dismal disappointment that when it's time for the bottom to fall out, it *does* fall out; they experience failure no matter what's happening.

In a more subtle kind of holding on, people grant that *something's* happened, some gains have been made, but nothing sufficiently major or magical. They suspect that they're missing out on the "flash" that everyone else enjoys, that the approach works better for everyone else than for them. This can be a simple crisis of confidence, a sign of self-doubt that refuses to believe that you can do what others can. Whatever results you get are automatically devalued because it's *you* who got them. Like Groucho Marx, who refused to belong to any club willing to accept a person like him as a member, you may be rejecting any technique that works for the likes of yourself. If so, adjust your estimate of success upward by twenty bonus confidence points (as you'd calibrate a meter that always read too low), and be sure to supplement your own evaluation with those of people whose judgment you trust. And start exploring the roots of your self-disparagement.

A particular distressing kind of holding on may make your symptoms seem worse. This, in fact, will happen to about 30 percent of patients at some time during treatment. When it does, you need courage to keep on persevering. Be reassured: this is a sign that the approach is working. Enough hidden feelings are stirring to arouse your symptom into a counterattack: you *are* having an impact; you've opened direct communication with the symptom. If these efforts can give you trouble, they can definitely take it away.

One last bit of holding on can be distressing far out of proportion to its impact. Some people find that the exercises have worked. Their symptoms have all but disappeared. But the last little patch of psoriasis will not go away; the herpes continues to recur, very mildly and occasionally; the warts that once covered your hand have left an enclave on the edge of one finger. The best thing you can do now is accept, even value this as a nostalgic souvenir of bad times, and a reminder of all you've done to help yourself. It's not a sign of failure but a last vestige of your experience, like the scar left by a disease or accident. You've domesticated what was once a wild beast, and you can take pleasure in living with something that once threatened and tormented you. Or think of it as a museum exhibit, preserved in a glass case, to be visited and pondered on a Sunday afternoon.

An important idea that reappears throughout this book is that we often get into trouble—including skin trouble—by replaying events and relationships of our long-ago past. As I've suggested here, such repetitions can throw up roadblocks to treatment. One particularly important kind of repetition, the relationship that develops between sufferers and those who are supposed to help them, is important enough for its own chapter.

19

Ghosts: Have They Handcuffed Your Doctors?

When skin patients come to see me, they have almost always been through a number of other doctors, from family physicians to superspecialists, in search of a cure. My role is often not to replace medical therapy but make it more effective—to remove barriers so my patients can benefit from their doctors' skills. This frequently means exorcising ghosts.

These ghosts inhabit the twilight zone of the mind, where past and present meet and mingle. They are the shadows of fathers, mothers, other all-important persons—*as they were experienced very early in life.* Just as unfinished business from childhood often generates or aggravates today's skin symptoms, these ghosts can intrude on, influence, even dominate today's relationships.

The technical term for the "ghost" effect is *transference,* and like resistance it has been studied extensively by psychotherapists. Freud noted early in his work that his patients *transferred* their childhood feelings about parents to him, and reacted to him as if he were the father or mother of long ago. He became convinced that transference could complicate therapy and raise resistance, but also generate insight and change. Transference makes it possible to reexperience the buried feelings of yesterday—openly and directly.[1]

Ghosts intrude into all our lives in familiar, minor ways: the new acquaintance or co-worker whom you like lavishly or resent unreasonably at first sight. You can often trace your reaction to the fact that he or she *reminds* you of someone from the past. You're actually reacting to your old girlfriend or your cousin Anne, not the personality of this person you hardly know.

Intimate relationships can be formed and destroyed under the influence of ghosts.

In the lives of people whose early years did not meet their needs, ghosts are likely to be particularly powerful. One person after another is cast as cold, withholding father or smothering mother, with the hope that this time they'll come through as they did not in the past. Like all efforts to rewrite history, it is doomed to fail.

Relationships with doctors are a fertile ground for ghosts. Your illness keeps you from full adult life, and as a patient, it's easy to fall into a childlike role—you're seeking help and protection from a person whose powers may seem larger than life. Many patients treat their doctors as little gods (and some doctors do little to discourage them), a relationship whose key precedent is the awe with which a small child regards Mommy and Daddy.

The conditions of treatment, too, encourage transference. The doctor is allowed to examine your body in an intimate, yet nonsexual way—the way your parents did when you were small. He or she may cause you pain, or instruct you to take medicine or follow procedures that are unpleasant or inconvenient—and you are expected to comply with these "doctor's orders" because they are *for your own good*, a line your parents may have used as they disciplined you.

David G., a computer engineer, came to see me after a series of dermatologists failed to relieve his multiple warts. He described how each doctor had used painful, difficult procedures (he spared no details) which sometimes brought temporary improvement. Then he concluded with a surprising note of triumph in his voice: "But they couldn't take them away!"

As details emerged, it became clear that for David, dermatology was a competitive game. If the doctor made the warts go away, the doctor won; if he failed, David won. It was more accurately a *no-win* situation.

We traced the roots of the game to David's father, who was

willing to give the young child the love and help he needed, but at a steep price: submission. When he joined young David for batting practice, for example, everything had to be done Dad's way; the boy was a virtual slave to his father during instruction. As usually happens, David went along on the surface, but his struggle for autonomy went underground. The ghost of Mr. G.—as the little boy experienced him—rose from the crypt of suppressed memory, clanked his chains, and turned a succession of adult relationships, including those failed attempts at treatment, into replays of *Life with Father*.

Here, the ghost phenomenon helped keep the symptom itself alive and recurring—the emotionally responsive warts appeared and persisted as David's minions in the fight for control. Ghosts may undercut treatment more subtly, too, making you "forget" to take medication or follow your doctor's advice—an indirect way to fight back against the ghost of a parent.

On the other hand, ghosts can prevent you from getting the treatment you need by demanding unreasonable loyalty. One of my patients remained for years under the care of a dermatologist who had been unable to rid him of persistent hives. He was hesitant to go elsewhere because this would seem a betrayal of the doctor, who after all was doing his best—an illogical persistence that made more sense as allegiance to the ghost of an idealized father.

Commonly, patients who go in and out of treatment with a series of doctors alternate between strong positive and negative feelings. They first cast the doctor as the Great Healer, larger than life, the superdoctor who will find the cure that no one else could. When he doesn't live up to his advance billing (what human being could?), the bubble bursts and disenchantment sets in. "The guy was so pompous—and it turned out he couldn't do a damned thing" is now the refrain.

The ghosts here may be of idealized, revered parents who didn't come through in fundamental ways, leaving their child persistently disappointed. Such was the story of Diane G. Her mother had been active in charity—a pillar of the community. Unfortunately, this left her little time or energy to give Diane the care and attention she needed. Suffering in adulthood with recurrent hives, Diane went through a series of doctors who seemed saints at first—like the public side of her mother—but who always let her down.

Just becoming aware that ghosts are complicating your treatment may help you evict them from what should be a helpful professional relationship. Once you recognize that you're dancing an old dance with your dermatologist, perhaps you can bring yourself to let go of it. If this particular relationship has become totally embroiled in unfinished emotional business, the decision to seek help elsewhere may be wise.

But to exorcise ghosts entirely from your treatment—as from other parts of your life—you'll have to come to grips with the unmet early needs that give them power. Like the "holding on" of the last chapter, ghosts can lead you to invaluable insights into the emotional tasks involved in your skin problems. They are not simply a wall, but a window into the deep parts of yourself.

It is often difficult to separate the clanking of ghosts' chains from your normal reaction to the real person—dermatologist, therapist, or whoever. But if you tune in to your feelings, you may note a kind of off-center, off-key quality, a sign that there's more here than meets the eye. A clue is *inappropriateness*. Are there times when your feelings about your doctor—about waiting in his waiting room, his appearance, his manner—seem mysteriously exaggerated or understated, as if you're actually reacting to something or someone who isn't there?

Ambivalence is another characteristic. Opposite, intense feelings often coexist when ghosts are involved. Do you feel that your dermatologist is Albert Schweitzer today, Dr. Caligari tomorrow? Such simple, intense reactions hark back to an era when all was black and white—the days of your childhood. Ambivalence can split in two, making you regard your dermatologist's nurse or receptionist as Ms. Hyde to his Dr. Jekyll.

"Ghostly" reactions are *tenacious*. In the normal course of relationships, our first impressions are softened and modified by subsequent experience. If your doctor first struck you as cool and formal, and you persist in thinking of him that way even though he's since warmed up considerably, consider the influence of ghosts.

We often defend ourselves against our ghosts with an exaggerated swing in the opposite, businesslike direction. If you find yourself playing a very neutral role with your doctor—a contrast to your usually expressive self—you may be trying hard to keep your ghosts from coming out of their crypts. This process may be operating in people who refer to their doctors as "plumbers" or "technicians," or who focus on the details of therapy to the exclusion of the human being who delivers it. If you're trying awfully hard to be a *good patient*, you may be holding down impulses and strong feelings the way children do when they're relentlessly good boys and good girls.

Ghosts can express themselves in action. If you find yourself arriving uncharacteristically late or compulsively early for appointments, or forgetting them altogether, your unconscious may be acting out fears and wishes that date from early relationships with parents. Similarly, it's appropriate to shower and dress carefully before visiting a person who will examine your body. But if you go through extended rituals, pay obsessive attention to cleanliness, and spend half the day deciding what underwear to wear, you should wonder *whom* you are really trying to impress, and in what way.

Sexual feelings that play an important role in skin disorders may also mark the work of ghosts. Do you cast the doctor as a glamorous, sexy person who refuses to notice you? Or a puritanical moralist who seems to disapprove of your sexual life, and of your body itself? If there is an element of exhibitionism, shame, or sexual fears in your skin problem, it may be most visible when you look at your feelings about your doctor.

Because the same ghosts remain in the background, there's often a repetitive quality to these relationships. Some people react to one doctor after another in the same way, or repeat patterns that also occur when they interact with such authority figures as bosses or teachers. The "ghost" may be an intermittent creature that periodically transforms an adult relationship into an echo of the past—usually at a critical juncture. Try to tap into repeated motifs and patterns that govern the ghost's appearances: this may open up discoveries about the emotional tasks that are haunting you.[2]

217

If you think ghosts may have stepped into your medical care, try the following exercise. Look back over the list of doctors you've seen for your problem. Describe each: simply write a list of adjectives, a paragraph, or just a word picture of disjointed phrases. Allow room for imagination. Don't worry if your descriptions are overstated—what we want is the *emotional* truth, the way the doctor seemed to you.

Add (if you can remember) a capsule description of your expectations, your first impression of each practitioner, your feelings about him or her after treatment. If someone other than the doctor became prominent in the course of treament—a nurse, a receptionist, the neighbor who gave you the doctor's name—include a description of him or her.

Now look over your lists and descriptions for recurring themes. Did these characters have something in common? Does this seem reminiscent of anything in your mother, father, or other key person in your early life? Often, ghosts are *triggered* by trivial details—a gesture, a tone of voice, a posture or quirk of expression. For mysterious reasons, these seem hard to take or utterly delightful. The explanation is the ghost that rises out of a small similarity.

A problem comes up if you feel that your reactions to certain doctors were strong—*but justified*. Drs. A., B., and C. *were* insensitive bastards; Dr. D. *did* promise things he couldn't deliver. Doctors are human beings and thus heir to the full range of foibles and frailties. If you feel that Dr. Z. treated you in an offhand, careless way, you may be right. At a particular time, a particular doctor may overreact, misperceive, be oversensitive or insensitive. (A patient may trigger something out of his or her past, for one thing. It is not uncommon for a cycle to develop involving both doctor's and patient's ghosts.)

There's no simple way to separate objective reality from ghost stories, and the real versus imaginary issue can pointlessly drain time and energy. So for the sake of argument, let's just assume that 50 percent of what you experience in your relationship with your doctor is objectively there, and 50 percent is the work of ghosts. Obviously, this won't correspond exactly to reality, but in the long run that doesn't matter. Just being open to the possibility that some of your reaction comes from within will clear the way to liberating insights. But certainly don't go too far and totally dismiss your criticism and reservations.

Take this opportunity to confront the issue squarely. If you feel you're being mistreated or shortchanged by your present doctor, bring it out into the open. If he or she is unwilling to discuss your feelings directly, you may have to find another doctor, but with such feelings festering beneath the surface, you probably wouldn't get much from this doctor anyway.

At the same time, allow yourself to *consider* that some of your problems with your doctor are the work of ghosts. What if his or her dereliction, disloyalty, disappointing behavior were simply not so? What if the similarities to past figures who bound you too tightly or let you go too brutally were imaginary? What difference would this make to your treatment? Have you dismissed advice that you might otherwise take to heart? Have you been persisting too long in a treatment that you'd otherwise examine critically?

GHOSTS IN PRINT

Although it's not as concrete as a person-to-person interaction, you've developed a "relationship" with me through this book. It may be as confusing—and revealing—as your relationship with your doctor. I've made demands, invitations, offers of help; tried to stir up your emotions and change how you look at yourself, your family, and your early life. Dealing with the emotions I've engaged can raise ghosts just as the transference of psychotherapy can.

Consider your enthusiasm or coolness toward the book, your irritation or hopeful longing. Am I a frustrating tease, dropping hints that are never followed up adequately? Do I promise more than I deliver?

What face do you see behind the voice that speaks these words to you? Does my tone convey seriousness, flippancy, concern? Am I a sincere, devoted healer? A pompous ass? Do you suspect that, underneath it all, I'm in it for the money, I'm directing your attention to your inner self so I can get my hand in your pocket? Am I well-meaning but misguided, or an adept professional? Am I a flaky Californian, a hard-headed New Yorker, a placid Mid-westerner—or a bit of all three?

Again, jot down adjectives, paint a word picture, or even sketch a literal picture of the "I" who has given you all this advice, instruction, and information. Write a one-paragraph review of the book—but a totally subjective, emotional review that conveys how you've experienced it, not how it might seem to a detached reviewer.

Go further and consider that this book is a collaboration combining the experience and intelligence of two people. Does your image split into extremes—the wise shrink and the cynical reporter? Do you attribute the book's strengths to one member of the team, its shortcomings to the other?

Imagine the process of collaboration: Grossbart and Sherman are sharing a six-pack, talking well into the night, working harmoniously with only the best interests of their book and its readers at heart. Or perhaps they sit at opposite ends of a cold copper wire, each at his word processer, or their disembodied voices twitter endlessly haggling on the telephone. Is their collaboration—a marriage of sorts—smooth or rocky? Do they have boundless appreciation for each other's skills and sensibilities? Do they respect each other's needs? Or hate each other's guts? Are they good parents to the "baby"—this book?

When you examine your feelings about the authors, their collaboration, and the book that has demanded your attention for days, weeks, or months, ask yourself the same questions you asked about your doctors. Have you ever dealt with someone like the author(s) before? Do your feelings now echo other feelings from other times? Is there a familiar quality in your frustration, your disappointment, your enthusiasm? Does your fantasy of their collaboration echo any other "marriage," any other "baby"? This exercise in introspection may help the book work better for you, as well as helping you know yourself. Once more, I urge you to look honestly and squarely at your feelings. They may not be logical or realistic (how could you know what the author is *really* like?), but they are *yours*.

PART FOUR

Disease Directory[1]

I often tell my patients not to focus narrrowly on the diagnostic label dermatology gives their skin problem. Your eczema or acne may be responding to the same needs, fears, and emotional tasks as your neighbor's psoriasis or hives. But I know that most people suspect that they have at least something in common with others who suffer the same rash or itch, and they want to know what my approach can offer *their* symptom or disease. Certain skin conditions can be associated with certain specific tasks, and respond best to certain techniques. Knowing this can foster insight and guide treatment.

For this section, I combed medical reports that have appeared in journals in a dozen languages over the last hundred years. The goal is to help you understand the emotional factors behind your particular disease; to answer the question "What will these techniques do for me?"

A few cautions:

• Science advances by generalizations, but you are an individual. What works for others might not work for you, and vice versa. Although "stopping the clock" is a common task behind adult acne, *your* acne may be "crying for love."

• The Griesemer index (see Chapter 5) gives only a rough, relative idea of each symptom's emotional responsiveness. If you are one of the 36 percent of herpes sufferers whose symptoms are worsened by emotional factors, *your* sensitivity is 100 percent.

• Because any persistent or severe skin problem has emotional impact, *any* skin patient with any disease can benefit from the techniques in this book. Even if emotional factors don't trigger or aggravate your problem, techniques like relaxation will make it easier to live inside your troubled skin.

If you can't find your symptom or illness here, ask your dermatologist for various ways it may be identified, or check one of the general references I cite. Often one skin condition goes under several different names.

ACNE

Griesemer index: 55%   Incubation period: two days

When the sebaceous glands begin producing their oily secretion just before adolescence, the common condition called acne frequently develops, with pimples, pustules, cysts, blackheads, even abscesses. Most acne, no matter how severe, disappears by the twenties, but the condition may persist or recur later in life. Most medical and proprietary treatments for acne are topical preparations using zinc oxide, benzoyl peroxide, antibiotics, and vitamin A derivatives. In moderate to severe cases, doctors often add antibiotics, usually tetracycline. *Accutane*, a medication related to vitamin A, is effective but must be handled with care.

There seems to be general agreement that stress can trigger and exacerbate adolescent acne, although the condition itself is basically physiological and hereditary. When acne outlasts adolescence, the importance of emotional issues increases, particularly conflicts surrounding growing up: the skin, quite literally, remains in adolescence.

The anguish of acne is unquestionable. Coming in the midst of the turmoil of adolescence, it can promote isolation, damage body image, provoke feelings of isolation, and impede sexual development. Acne sufferers frequently feel that their disease is "dirty" and makes them "repulsive." Many teenagers with severe acne can benefit from supportive psychotherapy and reassurance; an honest approach that recognizes and addresses teenagers' tendency to connect acne with guilt and punishment is critical. No tranquilizer can replace rapport and explanations that dispel fears and anxieties.

Psychological techniques that promote relaxation and reduce stress have proved valuable additions to medical therapy for acne. You may supplement these techniques with diagnostic work, aimed at exploring growing-up, stopping-the-clock, and sexuality issues that may heighten the symptom.[2]

ALLERGIES

Allergy is not a disease, but a mechanism that causes many diseases, including asthma and hay fever. Allergic skin eruptions follow exposure to plants or animals, or ingestion of food to which a person is sensitive. Such symptoms as hives and eczema are often caused by allergy.

These skin problems reflect a biological predisposition (probably involving the immune system), but psychological factors play a major role.

As the Japanese lacquer tree study cited earlier showed, an allergic reaction may follow exposure to a harmless substance to which a person believes he is sensitive. By the same token, an allergic reaction can be conditioned, linking a particular substance to an emotional issue.[3] One girl developed a strong allergic reaction to wood and wood products. When hypnotherapy allowed her to connect this to her difficult relationship with her father, who was a carpenter, the allergy vanished.[4]

These are just two of many research and treatment reports. I present more under the name of specific skin symptoms (such as hives or contact eczema). Hay fever and especially asthma are also very fertile ground for these approaches.[5]

ANGULAR CHEILOSIS

Ulcerations and cracks appear in the skin at the angles of the mouth, usually in connection with dental difficulties. Effective treatment requires dental correction of conditions that may cause drooling and skin irritation.

Secter and Batharthmi linked excess salivation to this symptom in one patient. She used her own self-hypnosis procedure—imagining her salivary glands to be a faucet, which she could adjust to maintain optimum flow—and focused on the disappearance of the lesions themselves, for noticeable improvement.[6]

BACTERIAL SKIN INFECTIONS (Furuncles [Boils], Folliculitis, Impetigo, Recurrent Infections, Pyoderma)

Griesemer index: 29%   Incubation period: days

Skin infections are usually treated with antibiotics and appropriate hygiene. Because the micrroorganisms responsible are for the most part ubiquitous, it seems that susceptibility to recurrent infections often involves a lapse in the body's own defenses. Emotional stress of various kinds is known to depress immune function, and many people have noted the appearance of boils or other infections at a time of turmoil.

Thus, any techniques that help you handle emotional conflict and defuse stress may have a beneficial effect on recurrent infections.

In one case, described by Jabush, hypnosis brought dramatic improvement where a host of other therapies had failed. The patient was a thirty-three-year-old man whose chronic condition of oozing boils dated back to his teenage years. By now, his body was covered with boils, furuncles, and scars. The organism responsible was known to be the common *Staphylococcus aureus*, but no medical treatment was effective. An emotional factor in his illness was suggested by the fact that the new boils appeared on his face after bad dreams and restless sleep.

Under hypnosis, the patient was told to imagine cold, tingling, and heaviness in the infected areas. He was instructed to use self-hypnosis and autogenics to relax and to extend the effect of hypnosis. His skin improved dramatically within a week, and continued to clear over thirty-three sessions.[7]

BALDNESS

The loss of hair that many men experience from their twenties onward is genetic and biological, and no psychological technique, medication, lotion, or cream can do a thing to retard the process.

Baldness itself is far less a problem than the response to it, which for some men is devastating and totally preoccupying.

227

One patient of mine, a South American agronomist with an international reputation, became preoccupied with the loss of his hair, counting the fallout in his brush daily and agonizing over the drain after each shower. For him, it became clear, the loss of hair represented the loss of potency: a bald man was a joke, a buffoon, and his slow transformation into such a person was understandably upsetting. In therapy, it became clear that these fears were linked to his father, a prominent politician held in high public esteem by his community, but in reality a tormented man addicted to painkilling drugs. To my patient, the loss of his hair signaled his own inexorable descent to his father's "degenerate" level.

When preoccupation with baldness—or any skin symptom or condition—becomes excessive, the cognitive techniques suggested in Chapter 14 are a good place to start, with psychotherapy as the next step.

BEHÇET'S SYNDROME

Recurrent ulcerations appear on the mouth, genitals, and sometimes the eye, where it threatens sight. Behçet's syndrome can affect other body systems: when the nervous system becomes involved, mortality is 50 percent.

The cause is unknown, but may be viral, hormonal, or immunological. There is no definitive medical treatment.

An emotional dimension to Behçet's syndrome was suggested by a study by Epstein and colleagues of ten patients. All had severe psychological problems, particularly excessive concern about bodily illness and aggressiveness, and difficulty dealing with anger. They had all suffered their initial symptoms and major relapses during emotionally critical periods—crises involving family deaths, job loss, hysterectomy, and economic setbacks. A recurrent theme in these crises was a relationship shift that forced the patient to take on a more or less grown-up role.

As a group, these patients were childlike and dependent on a parent or spouse. They had difficulty growing up and feeling like autonomous men and women. They were prone to severe depression.

A short series of three to four psychotherapy sessions was helpful to them.[8]

Chapter 7 may be a helpful exercise for Behçet's syndrome patients, with particular attention to feeding and sustenance issues surrounding the mouth, and sexuality when genitals are a focus.

In looking at the Time Line and other diagnostic exercises, be alert to tasks surrounding growing up, anger, and sex. With this potentially life-threatening illness, it is particularly essential to get down to serious emotional work—possibly with a therapist—as a possible deterrent to future recurrences.

BURNS

Burn is possibly the most painful assault on the skin. Not only is the original injury extremely painful, but therapeutic procedures applied along the long road to recovery are frequently agonizing as well.

Hypnosis and other psychological therapies have dramatically proved their value in controlling pain and easing the emotional trauma that accompanies serious burns. Studies have shown that hypnosis can reduce the need for painkilling medication. Children and adolescents seem to profit particularly, perhaps because of their generally superior trance capacity.

Psychotherapy to support and strengthen patients in their difficult passage back to health has proved effective by helping them mobilize their own coping abilities, focusing more on their resources and less on their liabilities. Group meetings for families are often a useful adjunct.[9]

CANCER
Griesemer index (for basal cell carcinoma): 0

The role of emotional factors in the development and course of cancer is one of the most controversial questions in the mind-body area. Very little has been written on skin cancer per se, but volumes have appeared advancing and attacking various hypotheses linking emotions, life history, and cancer.[10]

Some studies have connected depression and despair with a high risk of cancer. Others focus on the suppression of anger: malignancy, they say, is a biological result of repressed rage. Carl Simonton, M.D., described the cancer-prone personality as unforgiving, self-pitying, and resentful.[11] Because cancer typically takes years—even decades—to develop, it is difficult to link specific events to the disease, but trends have been noted. One study found, as a persistent pattern, the loss of a serious love object six to eighteen months before the diagnosis.[12]

G. Nicholas Rogentine at the National Cancer Institute tried to predict which patients with malignant melanoma (a particularly virulent skin cancer) were more likely to recover without relapse. He found that one question was a better predictor than all other social, medical, or personality factors: "How great an adjustment did your disease require of you?" Those who experienced the greater impact, who felt their feelings, were the healthy ones. Those who kept a "stiff upper lip" succumbed to the disease.[13]

Psychological techniques may be useful for skin cancer patients, if only to ameliorate the emotional impact of this disease. Skin cancer is not life-threatening in most of its forms, but the word "cancer" retains an exaggerated power to arouse terror, shame, and guilt. As for treatment, proper medical management may be augmented by techniques that promote relaxation and reduce anger and depression. Dr. Simonton has used imaging techniques against many forms of cancer, and anyone interested in them should read this book.[14]

CANKER SORES (Aphthous Stomatitis)

These painful sores appear recurrently on inner cheeks, lips, gums, tongue, and palate. They afflict 20 percent of the population, most commonly between the ages of ten and forty. Their cause is unknown, but recurrences have been linked to emotional and physical stress, premenstrual tension, injury, and fever. Emotional stress is the most commonly cited precipitant, particularly domestic, financial, and sexual problems.[15]

If you suffer from canker sores, use your Time Line to discover what, if any, stresses appear to trigger them. The most common tasks associated with this symptom involve difficulty growing up, expressing anger, and looking for love—but as in all symptoms, individual emotional links may differ.

Canker sores are often seasonal: worst in the winter and spring, better in summmer. Examine your own seasonal pattern for hints that will help you design an effective ideal imaginary environment.

DARIER-WHITE DISEASE (Keratosis Follicularis)

Genetic at least in part, this condition usually appears between the ages of ten and twenty. Blockage of sebum production causes pustular sores at hair follicles, palms, nails, and mucus membranes. There is risk of secondary infection.

One controversial theory connects Darier-White disease with vitamin A deficiency, and in fact ointments of vitamin A or its derivatives have proved effective for some.

A clinical report by C.A.S. Wink found hypnotherapy effective. A railroad worker had suffered recurrent pimples on his forehead, hands, and upper back since adolescence. It flared up when his wife cuckolded him, as happened periodically, and improved when she returned. After vitamin A and steroids had failed, hypnotherapy produced some improvement: the top of his left forearm improved noticeably within a week, as had been specifically suggested in the trance state. Further remission was achieved by having him return, in imagination, to the time before the symptom had appeared, when he was twelve years old. The results were then even more striking.[16]

Often, but not invariably, Darier-White disease follows a seasonal pattern: it improves in cooler weather and is worst in summer; sunlight in particular aggravates it. These facts may be helpful in designing an appropriate imaginary ideal environment.

DERMATITIS (Eczema)

Griesemer index: 52–76%   Incubation period: seconds to days

Eczema and dermatitis are interchangeable names for the same group of conditions—inflammations of the skin that may include redness, swelling, eruptions, oozing, crusting, and scaling. Itching, often severe, commonly accompanies eczema. There are five types of eczema—lichen simplex chronicus, atopic dermatitis, contact dermatitis, hand dermatitis, and nummular dermatitis.

Atopic dermatitis often appears early in life, but may arise at any time. Medical treatment includes environmental adjustments to minimize irritation; local creams and medications, including steroids; and antihistamines and phototherapy.

Many investigators have linked eczema to very early unsatisfied hunger for love and affection. Victims are often the children of anxious, undemonstrative, overprotective mothers who, often despite the best of intentions, cannot provide the stroking and cuddling that babies require to thrive.[17] Significantly, the rate of eczema is lower among breast-fed infants; the critical factor may be the cuddling and skin contact that accompanies nursing.[18] Along with the hunger for love, eczema patients frequently must deal with much anger, typically unconscious.[19]

I regard atopic eczema as a disease of two or more people, not just the patient himself or herself. The original relationship is usually mother and child; in adulthood, the same emotional turmoil is transferred to marriage, particularly one that revives the same issues of love and rejection.

No one profile fits all atopic eczema sufferers, but many are intensely active, compulsively driven people. They tend to be bright children who learn quickly and do well at school. Possibly, this striving personality type, like the eczema itself, represents a reaction to the insecure feeling of being unwanted and unloved.

The emotional impact of atopic eczema can be devastating. It can interfere with the stroking and fondling a young child needs to build a strong sense of self. The skin becomes the focus of attention and emotion to which all else becomes secondary: happiness, anger, sadness, joy are embodied in the scratching and treating of troubled skin, leaving little room for normal relationships with friends and family.[20] In adolescence, the pain and embarrassment of eczema interfere with normal relationships; focus on the pleasure and pain of scratching can disrupt the normal course of sexual development.

Because emotional issues are so central in the course and impact of atopic eczema, the whole range of psychological techniques are relevant. Psychotherapy and hypnosis, behaviorial techniques and biofeedback have all been used with documented success.[21] Be especially alert for certain tasks: "crying for love," "expressing anger," and "control." Material in Chapter 17 should be particularly helpful.

Nummular dermatitis (named for its coin-shaped pattern of skin lesions) is usually more troublesome in winter and may go into remission in summer: consider this in developing an ideal imaginary environment. One study documented a major role for emotional difficulties in this type of eczema: all exacerbations were linked to stressful events.

In *hand eczema (dyshidrotic eczema or pompholox)*, skin of the hand becomes dry, cracked and flaking. Victims are typically driven and self-critical, oppressed by a sense of failure and guilt. In some cases, the eczema follows compulsive behavior patterns: the "dishpan hands" of the fanatic housekeeper, and the cracked, desiccated skin of those whose compulsive cleanliness leads to constant handwashing.

A German study links dyshidrotic eczema to a struggle for autonomy—an attempt to "take one's life into one's own hands." Or an expression of the contrary feeling that "I can't handle this."[22] Military reports suggest that eczema of the hands and feet may express the wish to avoid marching to danger, or using the hands to kill.

Psychological techniques, including short- and long-term psychotherapy, hypnosis, psychoanalysis, behaviorial therapy, and biofeedback, have worked well.

Contact eczema would seem to be a straightforward matter of the body's response to noxious chemicals or plants, but in fact psychological factors are often important—as dramatized by Japanese studies (see Introduction).[23]

The course and treatment of contact dermatitis is complicated when occupational exposure is involved. Suspicion and fear
about noxious chemicals—quite justified by the American industrial tradition of disregard for workers' welfare—may lead to excessive handwashing, which aggravates any irritation. Workers'
compensation rewards continued illness and penalizes recovery.
Contact dermatitis is more prevalent where workers are dissatis-
fied and alienated, suggesting a combination of chemical and
psychological factors, and fast-spreading "pseudoepidemics" have
been known to take place.[24]

Lichen simplex chronicus occurs in circumscribed areas, and
Chapter 7 may prove useful in getting to its emotional roots. Obermeyer described a forty-year-old woman who developed a rash
on the nape of her neck: she had stilled her conscience, guilty
over an affair with a married man, by "putting it all in the back
of my head."[25]

Generally, the earlier eczema appears and the more widely it
spreads, the more work will be necessary for improvement. The
different kinds of eczema are among the problems that people
present to me most often. They have provded some of the most
gratifying applications of the techniques.

DIFFUSE HAIR LOSS (Telogen Effluvium)
Griesemer index: 55%   Incubation period: two to three weeks

In contrast to alopecia, in which hair loss is total or limited
to well-marked areas, hair is lost gradually and diffusely over the
entire head, or body. It resembles the hair loss that often comes
during pregnancy or two to four months after childbirth, or that
follows serious illness. The cause of telogen effluvium is unclear,
and there is no definitive medical treatment.

The process may be triggered by emotional stress. Kligman
has documented five cases in which hair was lost after profound,
severe strain. In one, a prisoner who had been tried for murder
and escaped conviction three times on technicalities was found
guilty at his fourth trial. After two months, he started to lose his
hair.[26]

Any psychological technique that addresses stress and personal turmoil are worth a trial for this condition.

HAIR LOSS (Alopecia Areata and Alopecia Totalis)

Griesemer index: 96% (for areata)   Incubation period: two weeks

A range of medical conditions can cause general or localized hair loss; in some cases, an immune defect appears to be part of this disorder.

Emotional factors are frequent. Wittkower and Russell found that patients with alopecia fell into three groups. Two-thirds had neurotic conflicts severe enough to warrant therapy; typically they were shy, inhibited and depressed. In one-fourth, hair loss had been triggered by a specific traumatic event. There was no clear-cut emotional problem or stress in the remaining group.[27]

Traumatic events that precipitate hair loss often involve threats to the person or those who are close to him. From the battlefields of World War I, for example, came reports of soldiers losing their hair during combat: one French soldier lost all his body hair within two weeks after a particularly vicious battle, and it did not return. (Often, however, hair grows back within several months after emotional pressure is relieved.)[28]

Among young children, Melman and Griesemer found a consistent pattern linking the loss of hair with other losses—particularly the loss of love. One child lost her hair rapidly after being abandoned by her parents; a nine-year-old lost her hair two weeks after a violent fight between her parents. Anger is often involved: they report a four-year-old boy who was enraged when people didn't give him things, and whose rage was followed by hair loss.

The same pattern may occur later in life. An eighteen-year-old man suffered sudden hair loss two weeks after calling a woman to make his first date; the anxiety of the dating game was probably less significant than his symbolic separation from childhood. Adult hair fallout often occurs against a background of sensitizing childhood loss.[29]

As for treatment, psychotherapy and hypnosis have been in-

235

consistent: they seem very helpful in some studies, of little use in others. My own experience has been encouraging. Alopecia often causes severe distress, and psychological therapies clearly have a role in its alleviation. Their impact in reversing actual hair loss is less certain.

HAIR PLUCKING (Trichotollomania)

Normal children pluck and pull their hair, in frustration, the same way they bite their nails and suck their thumbs. Excessive or persistent hair pulling may require a psychologist, not a dermatologist. When it starts later in life or continues past childhood, it is likely to represent more serious problems.

Typically, trichotollomania severe enough to require treatment is associated with the loss of love. One case history describes a twelve-year-old girl whose hair thinned noticeably when economic problems forced her to live apart from her family; when reunited, the situation improved. The birth of a baby brother, rejection by parents, illness of a sibling that absorbs all a parent's attention—all these have triggered hair pulling.[30]

Other case histories connect hair pulling with anger following an insult to self-esteem: one child began this behavior after having her hair cut short as a punishment.[31] A Japanese report by Oguchi and Miura suggests that a child who pulls his hair is acting on behalf of a troubled family: he is simply the "symptom bearer."[32]

The tasks most often connected to hair pulling are "crying for love," sexuality, and the expression of anger. Hypnotic techniques, including an adaptation of the "soothing hand" technique described in Chapter 17, may be particularly helpful.

In one case, psychotherapy alone did little for a twenty-six-year-old woman who compulsively and habitually pulled out her hair. But it was successfully combined with the hypnotic suggestion that she would become aware of her action as she reached for her hair, and this would make her scalp so sensitive that touching it would be painful.[33]

If you are dealing with a child who pulls her hair, you can be optimistic: simple behavior changes like providing more love

and attention may accomplish much—together with psychotherapy or hypnosis, if indicated.

HERPES SIMPLEX

Griesemer index: 36%   Incubation period: days

The herpes viruses are a large family responsible for a wide
range of diseases. The name comes from a Greek word meaning
"to creep," and reflects the observation that such infections often
creep or crawl across the body. Herpes viruses share the ability
to become latent—they retreat into hiding places in nerve cells,
and reappear weeks, months, or years later.

Herpes simplex infections are extremely widespread—perhaps more common than the common cold—and may occur anywhere on the skin and in a number of internal organs as well.
Fingers are a possible site, particularly among dentists and dental
hygienists; through skin contact, wrestlers can contract "herpes
gladitorium."

Oral herpes (cold sores; fever blisters) produces sores and blisters
around the mouth that are harmless to healthy people, but you
need to know how to avoid passing them on. Studies show that
half the people in the country have active outbreaks of oral herpes
at some time, and 70 to 90 percent have antibodies suggesting
that they have been exposed and harbor the virus with or without symptoms.

Like other herpes viruses, the agent that causes cold sores retreats to hide in nerve cells after the initial attack. Heat—sunlight or fever, for example—can trigger recurrences, along with
emotional turmoil. Flulike symptoms may precede or accompany
the first or later attacks. Although no medical treatment can prevent oral herpes recurrences, the condition is almost always self-
limiting. For the majority of people, recurrences grow shorter and
less frequent as the body becomes more adept in dealing with the
virus.[34]

The emotional responsiveness of oral herpes has been documented for decades. Over fifty years ago, researchers at the
University of Vienna used hypnosis to both alleviate and experimentally produce recurrences.[35]

In general, anything that promotes well-being and relaxation—such as the appropriate exercises here—may reduce the emotional pressures that trigger outbreaks. Get to know your personal triggers with the Time Line exercise, perhaps using a detailed log of events and recurrences.

This disorder has become less common over the years, but it has taken on a newly sinister meaning in the minds of many because of the hysteria surrounding genital herpes, which is caused by the same or a similar virus. Some people with oral herpes are sadly beginning to share the sense of badness and contamination that can afflict people with genital herpes. It helps to become aware of the needs, fears, and undone emotional tasks that may make you particularly vulnerable to feelings of shame, guilt, and dirtiness.

GENITAL HERPES (Herpes Genitalis)

Recent surveys indicate an 85 percent rate of recurrence triggered by emotional stress.

Sores and blisters appear on the thighs, buttocks, or genital region, and are usually transmitted sexually. Like cold sores, the lesions of genital herpes recur in some people but disappear spontaneously. In most cases, recurrences grow shorter and less frequent as the body learns to cope with the virus.

At this time, most medical treatment for genital herpes aims to reduce discomfort with analgesics, lotions, and baths. A recently developed drug, *acyclovir*, can shorten the duration of the initial infection and reduce length and frequency of the recurrence. Because the role of emotional turmoil in triggering outbreaks is well documented, psychological techniques are another effective means to prevent and shorten recurrences.

I think of genital herpes as three diseases: *medical herpes*, an infection caused by a virus; *psychological herpes*, the emotional impact of the disease; and *media herpes*, the burden of being a central character in a modern morality play, complete with the wages of sin, lepers and whores, and scarlet letters. Psychological techniques can offer much to anyone grappling with all three diseases. In fact, my work with herpes patients was a significant inspiration for this book.

A graphic demonstration of the pain of media and psychological vs. medical herpes was provided by a woman in my group who had been infected several years before, but who always dismissed the misdiagnosed outbreaks as nondescript and vaguely annoying. When her herpes was correctly diagnosed, however, she was plunged into turmoil and anguish.

Much preventable torment comes from misinformation about herpes. Myths and pseudofacts about complications, cancer, and pregnancy are widespread. As with any disease, facts are a key medicine: you need facts to decide what precautions will allow you to continue an active sexual life. A safe approach is holding off on intercourse from the first warning signs of a recurrence until after the sores have healed completely. Use contraceptive foam or jelly (they kill the virus) and condoms the rest of the time if you suspect a recurrence coming.

You also need facts and thought to decide what to say and when to say it to prospective and past sexual partners.

Women with herpes need to react but not overreact to a possible link with cervical cancer. Statistics suggest such a connection, but it is far from proved. Gynecological examinations and pap smears once or twice yearly will warn against this largely treatable cancer.

Ocular herpes does exist, and it is in fact the most common cause of blindness due to infection. But it is exceedingly rare, and virtually never occurs in connection with oral or genital recurrences. Precautions—don't touch your eyes after touching active sores; don't put contact lenses in your mouth if you have a cold sore—are worth observing, anyway.

Women with herpes understandably worry about its effect on pregnancy. An infant can indeed be infected by a mother who has an active genital lesion at the time of childbirth, but precautions will prevent this effectively. The important thing is making sure your obstetrician knows your medical history.

Because herpes is a fast-spreading disease involving the genitals and is recurrent, its psychological impact can be devastating. In a survey conducted by the Herpes Resource Center, 84 percent of people with herpes reported depression, 42 percent deep depression; 25 percent said they had self-destructive feelings; 35 percent reported diminished sexual drive and 10 percent withdrew totally from sexual involvements; and 70 percent reported a sense of isolation. Work performance suffered for 40 percent.[36]

Prominent among these emotional torments is a despairing sense of personal dirtiness or badness. "Outcast," "leper," and "whore" are frequent self-accusations. People with herpes are often filled with rage at the person who infected them. Some repress the feeling and torture themselves; some become cynical toward the opposite sex; a small percentage will even transmit the disease intentionally for revenge. A generalized feeling of alienation may lead some people with herpes to withdraw not only from sexual encounters, but from social interactions vital to good health: they cast themselves as pariahs and enter voluntary exile, feeding a self-destructive cycle of despair.

Such turmoil may markedly turn the course of the disease for the worse. Depression and other emotional upsets may impair the immune system that otherwise keeps the virus in check.

Anxiety about recurrences may *trigger* what is feared—a phenomenon I call "avalanching." When a *Time* cover story about herpes appeared, it aroused shame, anger, and anxiety in people with the disease—and a number of my patients suffered recurrences as a result.

Knowing that emotional turmoil triggers recurrences, people will unjustly torment themselves for feeling tormented. Similarly, people need to identify and reverse *agglomeration*, blaming the disease for everything wrong with their lives, including sexual problems, depression, and social withdrawal, that they may have needed help with even before they got herpes.

Not everyone with herpes reacts the same way, of course: like any disease, it affects you most strongly where you're most vulnerable—your emotional Achilles heel. The disease gets tangled up with unresolved issues that have lain beneath the surface since childhood, creating a double dose of turmoil.

In the case of herpes, it is particularly vital to ask yourself what the symptom is doing *for* you as well as *to* you. I can cite many instances where recurrences played the role of sexual policeman, inflicted self-punishment, resolved conflicts. A twenty-eight-year-old artist wanted to become a father, for example, but suffered a recurrence whenever his wife was fertile: clearly, the virus was acting on behalf of his doubts about parenthood. A twenty-six-year-old computer executive who harbored deep fears of intimacy endured recurrences whenever he met a woman who threatened to engage his affections by exciting him both sexually and emotionally. A religious forty-two-year-old advertising executive found herself drifting into an affair with a married man; she felt torn between passion and principle—until her herpes resolved her dilemma.

Biological factors help determine why some people never have herpes recurrences, while others have them almost ceaselessly: different strains of the virus are apparently more or less prone to recur. But it seems clear that for many people emotional factors are critical in determining the frequency and severity of recurrences, and psychological approaches offer an effective way to control the disease. In one study conducted at the University of Bologna in 1981, Dr. Arone Di Bertolino used hypnosis for nine patients who suffered genital herpes recurrences weekly or bi-monthly. One and a half months after treatment, six had no recurrences, three only one or two. Whenever new drugs are tried for herpes, the members of "placebo group" (who are given inert substances for contrast with those given the drug) usually enjoy some relief, demonstrating the mind's power to keep the virus in check.[37]

My own experience working with people individually and in groups has been extremely satisfying. In the group, we spent an hour and fifteen minutes doing psychotherapy aimed at exploring emotional tasks and life issues, then fifteen minutes going through exercises much like those in the book: relaxation, entering the hypnotic state and the ideal imaginary environment. Participants used the "soothing, healing hand" technique and also developed individual images of their immune system defeating the virus. Almost every participant rated the group helpful. Some set personal records for time between recurrences; others had the same number of outbreaks, but they were briefer and less severe; some learned to recognize prodromal symptoms and then to use the techniques to abort the full attack. Even when the disease didn't improve physically, people felt their new understanding helped them greatly to reduce its impact on their lives.

You can use many of these same techniques, relaxation, imaging, and hypnosis, to help short-circuit stress and encourage the body to a healthier state—possibly by enhancing immune function. Time Line and other diagnostic exercises will pinpoint your personal "herpes stress" that leads to the outbreaks. Diagnostic work can uncover emotional tasks like "sexual policeman," and "anger" that increase the number of attacks and their emotional impact.

You should contact the Herpes Resource Center (Box 100, Palo Alto, CA 94302). They provide educational programs, lobby for increased research funding, and sponsor a nationwide network of HELP support groups. Their newsletter *The Helper* is the ideal way to keep up on new research, practical hints, and opinions.

People with herpes have a growing number of good books readily available.[38] These are all worth reading, but I would particularly recommend the Langston book for both well-informed discussion of necessary medical facts and sensitivity to the psychological side of treatment.[39]

HERPES ZOSTER (Shingles)

Griesemer index: 36%   Incubation period: days

The chicken pox virus (one of the family of herpes viruses) doesn't die after an episode of that childhood disease, but retires to latency in nerve cells. Reactivated later in life, the same virus can cause the skin eruptions called shingles, which are often accompanied and followed by severe pain. Medical therapy for shingles (which accounts for 5 to 10 percent of all skin infections) aims at healing lesions and relieving pain. The use of steroids may reduce the incidence of post-herpetic pain, particularly in older patients. Experimental antiviral drugs look quite promising, as does AMP, a natural substance.

The factors that reactivate the chicken pox virus are complex, but depression of immune-system function plays a role. The immune system responds to depression and emotional trauma; stress and emotional turmoil are important in triggering and exacerbating shingles. Obermeyer cites a Czech paper that noted a high incidence of herpes zoster following psychic trauma, supporting my own observations.[40]

The pain of shingles can be excruciating, and hypnotherapy has proved itself most helpful here as in other painful conditions. Scott reports the case of a fifty-six-year-old man who went through years of drug therapy for shingles pain, nearly to the point of addiction, without lasting relief. Hypnotherapy to reduce pain directly was unsuccessful. In a dramatic use of the "making the symptom worse" technique (see Chapter 13), the therapist had his patient focus relentlessly on the pain, imagining it worse and worse until the merest brush of cotton on skin was unbearable. Under trance, the suggestion was made that the reverse was equally possible. After the second hypnotic session the patient could resume his golf games; at a reinforcement session eight months later, he suffered only slight pain—he was a changed man.[41]

HIVES (*Urticaria*)
Griesemer index: 68%   Incubation period: minutes

These raised, red, swollen spots on the skin affect 20 percent of the population some time. They often itch, sting, or prickle. Hives can be caused by a complex of physical and psychological factors: in children, allergy with possible emotional underpinnings is most common; in adults, emotional factors alone.

Medical reports describe one man who broke out in hives minutes after he'd been defrauded in a business deal! In a particularly interesting case of "pseudoallergy," a married woman ate lobster with her lover, in the course of a guilt-ridden affair. Thereafter, she developed hives whenever she ate lobster. Experimenters have experimentally produced hives by suggesting to subjects under hypnosis that they'd eaten food or come in contact with materials to which there were sensitive.[42]

Investigators such as Gloria Werth of George Washington

University Medical School emphasize the role of insoluble emotional dilemmas in recurrent hives. One patient, for example, was miserable in his job, but was reluctant to leave the city where his children lived with his ex-wife to seek another position. A young woman was resolved to remain a virgin until marriage, but found it hard to withstand her boyfriend's sexual importunities. An unmarried mother developed hives feeling trapped between her own aspirations and her responsibility to her child. A child felt forced to choose between warring parents.[43] If you suffer from recurrent hives, look for similar "hives dilemmas" in your own life.

Graham and Wolf of New York Hospital–Cornell Medical Center found a pervasive "hives attitude" among sufferers; they felt they'd been wronged or injured by a close family member, but couldn't retaliate or run away. Their skin showed physical signs of the emotional beating they'd taken.[44]

As a group, hives sufferers seem to have difficulty expressing anger: they may not permit themselves hostile or aggressive feelings or fantasies. Their need for love is often intense and can be traced back to a lack of parental, particularly maternal, love in childhood.[45]

Hypotherapy has proved effective for chronic hives. In one study, eighteen of twenty-seven patients had a complete or near complete recovery; eight others improved.[46] Short-term psychotherapy, behavior therapy, and relaxation have also given good results. In my own experience, a combination of psychotherapy with specific hypnotic techniques—the approach used in this book—has proved most effective.

HYPERHIDROSIS (Profuse Sweating)
Griesemer index: 100%   Incubation period: seconds

This increase in perspiration is usually in response to stressful or embarrassing situations. Since sweating is part of the fight-or-flight response and a bodily expression of anxiety, the emotional nature of this symptom is beyond question. However, profuse sweating can also be the symptom of a central nervous system disorder, so a good medical workup is essential.

Hyperhidrosis, whether confined to the palms and soles of the feet or more generalized, is distressing and embarrassing in itself. It can easily initiate a vicious cycle of "avalanching," in which fear of sweating triggers the unwanted response. If frequent and severe enough, it may promote secondary skin symptoms, including rashes, blisters, and infections.

Considering the major role of emotions in hyperhidrosis, and its emotional impact, relatively little has been written about psychological therapies for this condition. Many of the techniques described here can offer help for hyperhidrosis, particularly relaxation and self-hypnosis imaging techniques to reduce anxiety surrounding social and sexual encounters. The quick response to triggering events, characteristic of this disorder, should facilitate your diagnostic work and help you monitor your progress.[47]

ICHTHYOSIS (Fish Skin Disease)

In this hereditary condition, areas of the skin become dry and scaly, sometimes accompanied by severe itching. Doctors usually suggest environmental changes to keep the skin from drying out (emollient lotions, temperature and humidity control) and may prescribe steroid creams or vitamin A medications.

Ichthyosis is congenital, with no indication that emotions play a role in its origin. Yet hypnosis has produced striking improvements.[48]

Good hypnotic subjects enjoyed the most impressive results. One, a fifty-five-year-old man who imagined himself in a warm, comfortable imaginary ideal environment, achieved 45 percent improvement on parts of his body within one month, despite the cold weather that typically made his symptoms worse.[49] Where ichthyosis is widespread, therapists have successfully directed suggestions to one body part at a time. Generally, hypnosis and self-hypnosis help patients attain a more optimistic, active role in their treatment; in view of the importance of life-style in moderating symptoms, this can be critical.

INTERTRIGO

To treat this skin inflammation that appears in body folds, doctors often advise environmental changes that promote dryness, including light, absorbent natural-fiber clothing. Steroids and soothing lotions are helpful.

I haven't found any reports about psychological techniques in intertrigo itself. Hyperhidrosis can be a key aggravating factor, however, and when it is, techniques that reduce the anxiety that causes excess perspiration may be helpful.

LICHEN PLANUS

Griesemer index: 82%   Incubation period: days

Scaling pustules erupt on the genitalia and mucus membranes, often with severe itching. This condition, whose cause is unknown but may be viral or immunological, typically affects those aged thirty to sixty. Medical treatment uses topical and systemic steroids.

Chronic or triggering stress may play a role in this symptom, according to reports, but no specific emotional tasks seem to be prominent. The onset of lichen planus often follows anxiety over work: a reserved, stolid farmer developed the disorder after a period of intense worry about an impending foreclosure; an adolescent, after a change in work and personal relationships.

Hypnotherapy proved quite effective in one clinical trial: four of eight patients were cured, and three of the others experienced distinct improvement.[50]

LUPUS ERYTHEMATOSIS

There are two forms of lupus: a chronic discoid form that affects the skin only, and a severe systemic form that affects the whole body. The characteristic rash—raised, red eruptions, on face, ears, and scalp, followed by scaling and scarring—gives lupus its name, which suggests something gnawed by a wolf. Its cause is unknown, but the disease apparently involves the immune system and is at least in part hereditary. Medical treatment includes application of creams to isolated lesions, and oral drugs, such as steroids and chloroquine, for more widespread and severe disease.

Discoid lupus rarely becomes the severe systemic form, and is rarely fatal, but it can be quite disfiguring. It is a capricious disease, getting better and coming back spontaneously. Some doctors have noted the role of emotional stress in aggravating and triggering episodes: there's a clear link between chronic physical and emotional exhaustion and the onset of symptoms.[51]

If you have lupus, you may find the Time Line useful in identifying events and stresses that aggravate your illness. For physical relaxation, try self-hypnosis. Any of my techniques that help you deal with turmoil may prove a useful adjunct to medical treatment; exercises that explore emotional weak spots may help you handle the impact of the disease and its disfigurement.

MOLLUSCUM CONTAGIOSUM

This is a wartlike tumor caused by a virus. It may become inflamed and resemble a boil. Appearing on the genitals, it is a sexually transmitted disease. It is usually removed easily with cryotherapy (freezing), scraping, or electrodesiccation.

Suggestion and psychological techniques may be effective here, as they are with warts. An Italian paper by Di Bertolino reported success with psychological techniques with children.[52]

PERIORAL DERMATITIS

The cause of this condition, which involves reddening of skin and pustular eruptions around the mouth, is unknown. It primarily affects young women.

A German study found a predominance among highly motivated career women in their thirties.[53] Another study of eighty patients suggested a typical psychological profile: they had experienced severe childhood frustration; women in the group tended to perceive partners as idealized father figures, who disappointed them. The disease often appeared after failures in relationship or work.[54]

Psychotherapy has been used effectively in combination with conventional medical therapy. In one study, 90 percent of a group improved with treatment that combined psychotherapy and nonsteroid creams; 72 percent of these had previously been treated unsuccessfully with steroids.[55]

PRURITIS (Itching)
Griesemer index: 86%   Incubation period: seconds

This common symptom can occur with a wide variety of skin conditions, or alone. It can range in severity from a minor annoyance to a continual torture that dominates life. Itching is so important a symptom that I've devoted an entire chapter to it (Chapter 17).

PSORIASIS
Griesemer index: 62%   Incubation period: days

Heredity is clearly a factor in psoriasis; just as clearly, emotional factors play a role in triggering episodes and determining severity. Two to eight million people in the United States endure the scaling skin plaques of psoriasis, which may be limited to small areas or generalized over large parts of the body.

Five to 10 percent of psoriasis patients suffer an associated arthritis as well.

Photochemotherapy—a drug is administered, then followed by exposure to ultraviolet light—is often effective in psoriasis; steroids, tar pastes, and vitamin A derivatives (retinoids) are also used.

The role of emotional upsets in triggering psoriasis has been recognized for over a century in the Western world, and doctors in Persia described successful psychotherapy twelve centuries ago.[56] A variety of tasks and patterns may be involved, according to modern studies. English physician R. H. Sevile found that among sixty-two patients with psoriasis, the ones who did best were those who could identify stressful events that triggered their outbreaks: an understanding of provoking factors apparently improves, or at least accompanies, the ability to deal with the disease.[57]

The emotional impact of psoriasis in unquestionable. A study of a hundred long-term patients by Stanker noted that the majority considered embarrassment the worst feature of their disease. Stares, real or imagined, and fears of contagion among the uninformed took a substantial emotional toll. Indeed, ignorance of the true nature of psoriasis has long compounded its impact.[58] Only in 1809 was the disease distinguished from leprosy in Europe and America; in the Middle Ages, patients were declared dead by the church, or burned at the stake.

Readers in the British Isles can join the self-help groups offered by the Psoriasis Association (Northampton NN2 7JG, England) for support. American readers might consider organizing their own groups, if there are none at local hospitals.

Good results have been obtained with many of the techniques described here, including hypnosis, psychotherapy, relaxation, and biofeedback.[59] Warmth and sunlight improve affected skin for most (this is standard medical therapy) and should be considered in designing an ideal imaginary environment. Group psychotherapy has proved helpful to some patients, particularly in cushioning the impact of the disease.[60,61]

ROSACEA
Griesemer index: 94%   Incubation period: two days

This condition, which resembles perioral dermatitis, affects three times as many women as men, typically between the ages of thirty and fifty. It consists of persistent flushing, usually of the face, and an eruption that resembles acne. A particularly disfiguring form where the nose is enlarged and deformed (rhynophyma) is more common in men: W. C. Fields suffered from rhynophyma. Rosacea often responds well to antibiotics like tet-racycline.

It would be simplistic to call rosacea prolonged blushing, but some links between the symptom and the common experience are clearly present. Studies have found typical rosacea sufferers to be anxious and vulnerable to feelings of insecurity and inferiority, sensitive to criticism, easily discouraged, shy and socially ill at ease. Guilt and shame are commonly described by these patients. They seem unusually dependent on the good opinion of others.

Patients studied in depth often describe their disease as a punishment or a safeguard—suggesting the importance of the "anger" and "skin as policeman" task. Another repeated theme is having to grow up prematurely, possibly due to the inadequacy or death of a parent or economic hardship. Social or sexual stress often triggers exacerbations.[62]

An attempt to explore underlying emotional factors and a method to modify your response to stressful situations (such as relaxation or hypnosis) are clearly worth a trial in resistant rosacea. Scott described one case in which a woman suffered an eruption of rosacea shortly after the death of a close friend. On the surface, the patient showed little grief; in hypnosis, it was clear that her grief had been stopped by intense jealousy of her more attractive friend, who had stolen her boyfriends in the past. Improvement followed quickly after this issue was out in the open, showing how responsive this symptom may sometimes be.[63]

SEBORRHEIC DERMATITIS

Griesemer index: 41%   Incubation period: days

In this condition, which resembles dandruff, accelerated growth of skin cells produces red, scaly eruptions. Medical treatment aims to eliminate scaling with shampoos using selenium sulfide, zinc pyrithione, and tar.

There has been little research into emotional factors that may trigger or follow seborrheic dermatitis. Witkauer and Russell found that two-thirds of one hundred patients experienced social difficulty: they feared ridicule, or simply being conspicuous. As a group, they were slow to make friends, hardworking, and perfectionistic. Almost all described triggering incidents that threatened their self-esteem.[64]

The techniques I've described may work in seborrheic dermatitis; but here more than with many other conditions, you must be your own researcher.

SELF-INFLICTED WOUNDS (*Factitia*)

Griesemer index: 69% Incubation period: seconds

People inflict a wide variety of wounds on their skin—tearing, cutting, freezing, burning themselves. The wounds may be treated by a physician, but their cause is clearly psychological, and requires an appropropriate approach.

You don't have to be crazy to damage your own skin, although some such self-victims are in fact psychotic. Most are simply acting out in a particularly concrete way the kind of self-destructive impulses that others do more subtly. There are ways in which virtually all human beings treat themselves poorly—they range from the extreme of suicide to self-defeating behavior: ("fractional suicides") like self-isolation, self-neglect, poor diet, and failure to take medication when indicated.

If you inflict damage to your own skin, don't feel like a freak—what you're doing is a dramatic expression of a near-universal mechanism—but do make a determined effort to get to the bottom of your symptom. The first step is owning up to the action and taking responsibility for it—and regarding yourself and your trouble with the same compassion you'd have for a friend. Shame and humiliation are a natural response, but are neither necessary nor helpful. Why flagellate yourself for something you cannot, as yet, fully control?

This advice is also directed to anyone who in any way aggravates a skin symptom, by picking or squeezing pimples, compulsively washing hands plagued by dry skin, or rubbing places that are already irritated. Only when you take responsibility for what you're doing can you become an active party in helping yourself.

Any and all the exercises in this book may help you gain insight into the tasks that your skin assaults are seeking to accomplish. Anger, love, sexuality tasks are likely to be particularly relevant. Self-damage is always a cry for help. It may attempt to atone for an obscure sense of sin: some people report that they damage their skin with a feeling of purifying themselves, of releasing enormous pressure. It may seem the only way to get special care and nurturance, particularly for those whose parents came through only in times of illness or distress.

Don't overlook loyalty as a motive for self-destructive acts. Anyone who treats himself badly was *taught* to: often we take over the task of chastising ourselves to keep up the work of physically or emotionally abusive parents.

Because the emotional nature of this symptom is particularly difficult to grapple with alone, be particularly ready to seek professional help.[65]

STIGMATA AND SPONTANEOUS PURPURA

Stigmata are marks that appear spontaneously, usually duplicating the wounds of Christ: bruises may appear on the forehead, suggesting the crown of thorns; stripes on the back, indicating the weight of the cross; and wide plaques on the hands, corresponding to the nails of crucifixion. However, they also appear in members of other religions—Mohammedans while contemplating the battle wounds of Mohammed, for example—and in the nonreligious. Their cause is unknown, and there is no medical treatment. They're a striking example of the interaction of mind and skin.

Perhaps related are spontaneous purpura, or hemorrhages beneath the skin, which often appear after violent dreams or hallucinations. Victims are predominantly female and usually involved in some sort of emotional turmoil; the phenomenon is most likely to occur in the highly suggestible.

Hypnosis and psychotherapy may help in these conditions. In one woman, pains of the hands and feet, which appeared while she was contemplating the crucifix, disappeared with the help of hypnosis.[66]

VITILIGO

Grisemer index: 33%   Incubation period: two-three weeks.

The cause of this disorder, in which areas of the skin completely lose their normal pigmentation, is unknown, but the immune system may play a role. Psoralen compounds are often used to repigment the skin, bleaching of surrounding skin to blur the margin of the lesion, and stains or cosmetics to cover it.

Vitiligo causes no pain, physical discomfort or disability: it is purely a cosmetic condition. But as such it causes extreme distress. In one study, two-thirds of patients with vitiligo reported embarrassment; one-half said they were socially ill at ease, felt ugly or dressed inappropriately to hide affected areas. Over one-third said it interfered with their sex life. Two-thirds reported that strangers stared at them, 72 percent said they asked questions, and 16 percent said they made rude remarks. A full forty percent appeared to be chronically depressed by their symptom: "I hate myself; I feel like a freak" were typical comments.

Higher self-esteem and ego strength characterized patients who coped best with the burden of vitiligo. It appears that a person who generally feels better about himself or herself will better handle the self-image assault and embarrassment of this condition.

One complaint that emerged in patients' reports was their doctors' insensitivity to their needs and problems; they felt they needed more personal interest, encouragement and support.[67] A patient with vitiligo who feels this way might reflect that those needs are absolutely legitimate, but the dermatologist may be ill-equipped, by training and temperament, to satisfy them: psychotherapy can better provide support and foster adjustment to the disease.

One case history reports striking success against vitiligo with hypnotherapy. A. K. Gajwani, D.P.M., of Goa, India, described a twenty-seven-year-old woman who had an irregularly pigmented area near the left edge of her mouth, for seven years. (In India, the author notes, vitiligo carries a dire social stigma.) She lived in a strained situation with her in-laws and an unsatisfactory relationship with her husband, whose business activities kept him from devoting much attention to her.

In six sessions of hypnosis (at which she proved adept), it was suggested that her face was flushing and the white spots getting smaller. By the third session, the area had shrunk to half its original size. By the sixth, it had disappeared completely. On doctor's advice, her husband spent more time with her, following a "prescription" for movies, picnics, and walks. At follow-up, she appeared perfectly healthy.[68]

Generally the fact that emotions play a triggering role in one-third of vitiligo suggests that hypnosis and other psychological therapies may be helpful.

WARTS

Griesemer index (multiple, spreading warts): 95%   Incubation period: days

Warts are benign skin tumors caused by viruses. They are common, particularly between the ages of twelve and sixteen (a British survey found them in 16.2 percent of schoolchildren),[69] and usually removed easily by such dermatological procedures as electrocautery and cryosurgery (freezing). When they recur and spread widely, however, they can be extremely troublesome.

The treatment of warts is the area where psychological techniques have made the greatest inroads into the mainstream of dermatology. Warts seem to disappear and return spontaneously, but their behavior is often linked to emotional factors. The critical factor may be the immune system, which keeps the virus in check or allows it to flourish.

Human beings have long exploited the emotional sensitivity of warts with a huge arsenal of folk cures. Toads have been sacrificed, cats brought to graveyards at midnight, rituals performed, and incantations sung in efforts to make these growths disappear. There's substantial evidence that such cures work, beyond the spontaneous remission rate.[70]

Warts often respond dramatically to simple suggestion; as mentioned, I've had patients report their disappearance after calling me for an initial appointment. Laboratory investigations and clinical trials have shown hypnosis, in particular, to be effective.[71] One group of children, under treatment for other diseases with drugs that suppressed their immune system, were vulnerable to warts that resisted medical treatment. Even here, hypnosis was successful, with the better hypnotic subjects enjoying the best results.

Dr. Owen Robbins described a young boy who was plagued by severe recurrent warts—and a difficult family situation. His skin cleared quickly after he performed the overdue act of punching his intrusive, overbearing younger brother.[72] I've been impressed how often warts become a problem for people who are deadlocked in an emotional crisis, a stalemate that must be resolved for life to continue, or a general impasse in the process of growing up.

The most effective psychological approach to warts combines hypnotic techniques with exploration of troublesome issues, focused on today's impasse. With insight and life changes that release the patient from his emotional bind, the prognosis, even when warts are severe, is good. Rapport with a doctor who sincerely believes in these techniques is essential. Severe recurrent warts are one of the most frequent reasons people come to see me. Results are particularly favorable.

GENITAL WARTS (Condyloma Acuminata)

These have special emotional impact because of the area where they appear—the genitals and around the anus. Unlike other warts, they are contagious, with growing evidence suggesting links to cancer.

These warts often play the role of sexual policeman. They orchestrated one patient's ambivalence between his wife and girlfriend: whenever he was ready to return home, warts on his penis flared up and made his wife reluctant to take him back. With the hypnotic suggestion that he handle the situation directly, the warts vanished within three weeks. A twenty-seven-year-old insurance adjuster suffered from anal warts—and a fear of anal intercourse. Once he accepted the fact that he was in control—no one would subject him to anal rape, so the warts were unnecessary—they vanished in two sessions.[73]

Most people with warts find an ideal imaginary environment that incorporates cooling, and perhaps tingling, to be helpful, along with direct suggestions that they disappear. If these measures don't work, try to understand and clear away any possible emotional impasse: headway here often allows hypnotic techniques to become effective.

APPENDIX I:
One Woman's
Story (A Struggle)

[I've never met the woman from San Francisco who described her successful struggle against severe early eczema in the following story; she contacted me after reading my *Psychology Today* article. I often give copies of her story to my patients. We are grateful for her help.]

My history with eczema can be broken down like this: scratching and crying: infancy to age five; scratching and praying: age five to eight; physical attempts to control scratching; age eight to eleven; the psychological approach that saved me: age eleven to fourteen.

Until recently, I'd never heard the word "excoriation," but now I know it was my primary symptom: "scratching so severe as to tear the flesh." That's what I did every night, clawing till blood flowed. I was shocked to read that neurotic excoriation is caused by emotional difficulties 98 percent of the time. I was taken to doctor after doctor from 1957 to 1971, but this was never mentioned: no one acknowledged that I had emotional problems. Perhaps my parents thought the problems would go away if they pretended they weren't there. Maybe they were ashamed to admit their daughter might have such problems.

I *was* told that stress aggravated my condition, but only when I verbalized my anger, fear, and worry: "Stress aggravates your skin, honey—try not to think about those things if they upset you," they said. Actually, I couldn't express the many things that upset me, and I took out my frustration on my skin. I was desperate for explanations and reassurances. I was always depressed: I believed I was doomed to a life of hell on earth.

Because my skin condition developed at such an early age, it became as much a part of my identity as my brown eyes. I was always conscious of my parents' anxiety about me, and other people's reactions to my appearance. I imagined myself a martyr for an unknown cause.

Nighttime was the hardest time. Without the day's distractions, it was just me and my itching, me and my skin. Kids with severe eczema have an early self-awareness that comes from confronting themselves in the dark every night. The nightmare is your own body; the monster is you. This is emotionally devastating to a child because it breeds self-hatred; when you feel so bad, you think you must *be* very bad—what did you do that you're being punished for? Parents' reassurances are dwarfed by the power of the itch, like an evil spirit. It was basically a solitary struggle.

At age eight I was fascinated by Houdini because he had been able to escape any physical confinement—handcuffs, straitjackets, chains. I myself was put into straitjackets, handcuffs, chains, and gloves to keep me from ripping my skin to shreds every night. I would spend my nights figuring ways out of confinement; I'd wriggle my skinned and bleeding wrists out of the cuffs and tear at my flesh with a sense of triumph.

Eventually I learned to stop myself from scratching by concentration: I tucked my hands under my butt and pretended they were paralyzed. But whether I struggled to free myself to scratch or to stop myself from scratching, I would only strive for a harsh physical control over my body. For three years I was a wild animal with myself as prey.

I was a secretive child, always ashamed of my skin. Trying to hide, to pretend I was normal, to fool everyone by remaining mysterious, I lived in a fantasy world, I hated to explain my allergies: I told all sorts of lies, believing no one would go near me if they knew the truth. I became cynical at a very young age, hardening myself after so many disappointments: the doctors promising miracle cures, my parents promising miracles from God.

Looking back, I can see the sexual side of my eczema. I was able to touch and play with my body more openly than most children; strangers were always peering at and touching my naked body. I needed to have oils and lotions rubbed all over me, a task I particularly enjoyed when performed by my father: he gave me a good workout with his big, muscular hands.

Scratching was like ecstasy to me: digging my nails in and running them up and down my body was orgasmic; I moaned and grunted as I scratched and clawed myself.

I can remember the advantages. Everyone gave me and my skin attention: it made me important, although in a negative way. I got sympathy and affection that other kids didn't get. It was a way to miss school, sleep late, be lazy and spoiled, feel special and unique, spend time alone and in fantasy, avoid social confrontations.

My situation was painful, but it was safe and familiar, keeping me dependent and afraid of risks. I always had an excuse to avoid an unwanted task—I was the exception to every rule.

Before age eleven, I believed a fierce vigilance the only defense against the all-powerful itch. The only relaxation I remember from those years was exhausted collapse after scratching myself into a frenzy. But then I learned to relax consciously.

This came about through my attempts to overcome my insomnia. Left to themselves, my hands would scratch automatically, and it was scratching that kept me awake. To keep my hands otherwise occupied, I held them up in front of me and touched the fingertips together one by one, watching them slowly move and lightly touch, thumb to thumb, forefinger to forefinger, down the row and back again. In this way I hypnotized myself to sleep.

After a while I realized that this not only helped me sleep, it lessened my desire to scratch. I wasn't *forcing* myself not to scratch; I just didn't *need* to. I was overjoyed with this new feeling: for once, I would let go of my vigilance and still feel safe. I then observed that my slow, deep breathing during this little exercise was in itself enough to relax me; soon, whenever I sensed a wave of fitful scratching approach, I'd close my eyes and breathe deeply to break the chain reaction.

I learned to defuse triggering situations. For example, if I exercised or got nervous to the point of sweating, I'd start scratching wildly. I believed I was allergic to my own sweat, and I convinced the doctors that I should be excused from gym class for this reason.

Then I developed an alternative. When I started to sweat, I'd relax by deep breathing and tell myself: "You don't feel any itch. Your skin is fine. Sweating is okay. You don't have to scratch when you sweat. Just relax, sit quietly until you stop sweating, and you'll be fine." With my relaxing and soothing self-talk, not only didn't I itch, but the redness, welts, and hives that often accompanied sweating no longer appeared.

I learned to ignore the itch and my ravaged skin, leaving it to heal in peace. After years of ripping scabs off partially healed gashes and clawing them open to bleed and deepen, I finally learned to enjoy watching wounds heal.

I became able to limit my scratching to circumscribed areas. I'd allow myself to scratch my legs, for example, as long as I left the rest of my body alone. Then I gradually reduced the permissible area until there was no place left to scratch. Or I'd first let myself scratch my arms, narrow that down to the hands, then to one finger. For some time, I had my scratching narrowed down to my lower legs, which I continued to use as a battleground. Since last year, however, I've been totally free of rashes, wounds, and itching. I've let the hair grow on my legs to seal that "tomb" forever.

Before, my hands had been the enemy, inflicting rape and torture on my innocent body. I hated them. Once I learned to relax, I made peace with my hands, treating them with the same tenderness and respect I wanted them to show my body. I learned to use them for healing. Saying, "What do you really want, skin?" I'd stroke the damaged, itchy areas, kissing them and rocking as I hugged myself.

I learned to communicate with myself, talking out loud. At first, I told myself stories to distract myself from scratching. Then I learned how to tell myself what I needed to hear. I would pretend I was my mother telling me that she loved me; then I'd speak in my own voice, saying how afraid I was that I'd never get better. And on and on, taking turns with voices until I'd said all I needed to say and hear. As I hugged and stroked myself I'd cry and assure myself, "Don't worry, I'll take care of you," creating my own support system for changing my life.

I began to tell myself—and believe—that I was doing my best at every moment: if I couldn't control myself this time, I'd do better next time. "Can I stop scratching now?" I'd say. "If I can, that would be good. If not, that's okay too—I'll give myself five more minutes to scratch, and then stop. But next time I won't have to scratch at all." I gave myself high praise when I didn't scratch. The praise, I knew, had to come from myself, since I no longer believed anyone else. I congratulated myself for keeping clear what areas of skin I could.

When I decided that I, not my parents or my doctors, was my own savior, I stopped worrying about other people's infuriating questions, their warnings about scars and their promises of miracles. I stopped worrying about looking ugly or causing a public scene by scratching when I needed to scratch. No longer ashamed of my uninhibited self, I started answering questions frankly and addressing people's fears of contagion matter-of-factly.

I saw that I had a right to handle my disease in my own way, whether or not it was offensive to others. I claimed my right to be treated with respect, not like a leper or an uncontrollable child. I developed the confidence to go out in public, whether or not my skin was beautiful. I finally realized that no one was scrutinizing every pore of my skin—and that even if they were, it was none of their business and I was not obligated to look good for them.

I learned not to fear my emotions, gradually understanding how to deal with them calmly instead of falling, in an overwhelmed panic, into a chain reaction of scratching. Listening to my deepest instincts, developing a relationship with myself based on love, respect, and communication, I experienced a rebirth.

APPENDIX II:
Seeking Professional Help

In an ideal world, you'd find a great wise healer to help you get well—an expert in dermatology who understands psychotherapy and is adept at hypnosis. But in reality, Superdoctor is a mythical being, a cousin of that cartoon hero who appears in times of great need. This book is dedicated to the truth that you must take an active role in restoring and maintaining your health—which may mean recruiting your own *team* of professionals, including a physician and psychotherapist. Be ready to educate your dermatologist about the psychological side of your disease, and to explain your skin disease to an otherwise knowledgeable psychotherapist.

CHOOSING A DERMATOLOGIST

I urge you again not to start work with this book before seeing a competent medical specialist. This probably means a dermatologist (for some conditions, an allergist, urologist, or gynecologist). How to find one? A referral from your regular family doctor or internist is customary; or inquire at a local clinic or hospital. Perhaps a friend can recommend a doctor. Lists from the state medical society or professional society are helpful, but they won't tell you much about the quality of different practitioners.

There are three things to look for in a dermatologist (or any doctor whose help you enlist), but only one is essential: *technical competence. Sensitivity* to the psychological side of skin disorders is helpful, but the fact is that many highly skilled practitioners simply don't speak psychological "language." If your dermatologist feels there's no emotional side to your problem yet you feel there is, believe your hunch—and keep him on your treatment team. Thirdly, most of us seek a doctor who is "our kind of person," who *shares our basic values and prejudices.* Find one if you can, but remember that a skilled skin technician can help you get well even if he isn't someone you'd choose for a friend.

Many people come to me after seeing several, even several dozen dermatologists, each of whom has been disappointing. If this has been your experience, don't swear off medical care forever, but find a state-of-the-art specialist. (This will probably require a trip to a major teaching hospital or medical center, perhaps in a larger city.) A senior consulting dermatologist may or may not give you the results you seek, but at least he or she will get you off the merry-go-round cycle of "maybe the next will be better." And reread Chapter 19 for clues about personal problems that may make it difficult to find the right doctor.

GETTING PSYCHOLOGICAL HELP

Many people are still uncomfortable seeking help for emotional problems. Counseling for a difficult child or expert care for a serious mental illness sounds perfectly reasonable, but they feel that basically healthy adults should be able to work things out on their own. Seeking help appears to them a sign of weakness. If you feel this way, reread Chapter 16 for a realistic perspective.

Even if you're ready to seek help, it may not be easy to find a good psychotherapist. Expect to expend energy for a two-step process: finding a referral source, then finding the therapist you'll actually work with.

Your physician or clergyman may know of a good psychologist, psychiatrist, or social worker, or friends may have suggestions based on their own experience. Some cities have referral agencies that perform this "matchmaking" service for a small fee. Most mental health facilities—clinics, Community Mental Health Centers, and the like—maintain lists of staff members who have therapy time available.

Several published sources list mental health practitioners in your area. *The National Register of Health Service Providers in Psychology* is available at most good libraries, along with similar rosters of psychiatrists and social workers; these indicate formal credentials as well as areas of specialization.

Consider whether you'd prefer to work with a male or female, older or younger therapist. There are numerous schools of therapy, each with its own approach, and you may wonder which will suit you best. Your experience with this book may help you describe to a prospective therapist what approach you're looking for. You needn't know gestalt from deconditioning to tell him or her: "When I started looking at how my mother treated me as a child, I felt I was close to understanding something fundamental about my skin," or "I just want someone to coach me on relaxation techniques."

Interest in and experience with mind-body problems are a definite plus, but don't hold out till you find a skin expert—very few therapists have that orientation. Trust your instincts: someone who seems tuned in to your problem probably is. But if things just don't click, don't hesitate to look elsewhere.

If you've gone through three or four therapists without feeling heard and understood, consider that this difficulty may be part of your problem, and that rapport may come as therapy progresses. (Note to people with genital herpes: local HELP groups often have lists of helpful therapists.)

SPECIALIZED TECHNIQUES—RELAXATION AND HYPNOSIS

Many people with varied qualifications offer instruction on relaxation, and practice hypnosis. You're best off working with someone with mental health credentials: a psychologist, social worker, or psychiatrist who's received additional training in these techniques. Two highly reputable professional groups publish directories of qualified hypnotherapists: the Society for Clinical and Experimental Hypnosis, and the American Institute of Hypnosis.

PAYMENT

Health insurance has made psychotherapy a practical possibility for many. Check your policy (you may have to call the company for clarification) to answer three key questions: Does insurance pay for outpatient mental health services? Which therapists does it pay? How much does it pay?

Your policy may pay for psychotherapy, but not hypnosis, biofeedback, or relaxation, because these are considered "experimental techniques." (Often you'll be reimbursed if these techniques are billed under the general heading "psychotherapy.") It may pay for therapy performed by a psychiatrist or psychologist, but not a clinical social worker. It may insist that you be referrred by a physician.

Most policies have a yearly or per-session limit on coverage, and some exclude many problems as "preexisting conditions." If psychotherapy is not covered or inadequately reimbursed and finances threaten to become a hardship, consider therapy at a clinic or mental health center with a sliding scale based on your income. Group therapy is less expensive and in some cases more useful than individual sessions.

APPENDIX III:
If Your Child Has
the Problem

People with particularly short memories may believe that childhood is an idyllic, stress-free land, but surely most of us can see through that myth.[1] Children may not worry about fixing the roof and paying taxes, but they have strains and anxieties of their own, no less tormenting than grownups', which play as significant a role in their skin disorders. By the same token, nearly all my exercises can be translated into child-sized versions. Children, in fact, are particularly adept at diagnostic and treatment exercises. They respond better than adults who have suffered with resistant skin problems for years.[2]

As the parent of a child with problem skin, you are in a frustrating situation. You may wish you could take on your child's pain as your own, and stand willing to make any sacrifice, but you know of nothing you can do beyond taking him or her to the best doctor available.

Your feelings may be complicated by a vague sense that you are to blame: that your child's skin is a silent indictment of your parenting efforts. Let's face the issue squarely: what's needed is responsibility without self-flagellating guilt. Every parent does the best job he or she can. Many of us, however, simply cannot be as good parents as we'd want to be—economics, personal crises, pressing emotional problems of our own get in the way—and such difficulties can contribute to a wide range of skin problems.

266

Better to accentuate the positive: you are in a powerful position to help your child by understanding his or her emotional needs, searching for the roots of problems under the skin, perhaps bringing him or her the benefits of relaxation and self-hypnosis, with this book as a guide.

One key notion to remember is that children's skin conditions are often triggered or exacerbated by a *normal crisis*, an unavoidably stressful family event such as the birth of a sibling, relocation, the arrival of puberty, or a death in the family. Use the Time Line of Chapter 5 to see what was happening when the trouble started, and to pinpoint significant emotional issues.

Also keep in mind that working with your child on his or her skin problems is different at different ages. For the infant or small child who has not yet learned to talk, it's really yourself you must work on. Whatever helps you feel open, relaxed, and good about yourself also helps your child. If your needs aren't being satisfied, you won't be able to provide the rocking, soothing, stroking, and singing that your child and his skin need. Get the help *you* need, whether this means a laundry service, child guidance, or psychotherapy.

Can you act as a therapist for an older child? There's no simple yes or no. You might mention to your child that you've been reading a book about skin problems—like his or hers—and some games in the book sometimes help make troubled skin better. Many children really enjoy filling the Time Line and puzzling over "Why there?" (Chapter 7)—to say nothing of the Animal Test (Chapter 4). Keep the tone light but serious—you're working together on a puzzle or mystery. Don't push a hesitant child, and avoid pressured approaches (like the relentless "What if it got worse?" exercise of Chapter 10).

You might share the Benson relaxation technique (Chapter 11) with your child, and then work out childhood versions of exercises like the ideal imaginary environment (Chapter 12). Most children are adept at this sort of game, once they're ready to do it. (One hint: a lot of youngsters prefer to keep their eyes open, since closing their eyes reminds them of going to bed.)

The woman who tells her story of triumph over eczema in Appendix I also had some important observations, based on her own experience, about how parents can help their children. She's talking specifically about eczema, but much applies to other skin conditions as well:

> Kids with eczema need extra indulgence at bedtime. During bad periods, parents may need to lie down next to the child until he or she falls asleep, then go back in the middle of the night to help him or her fall asleep again. Singing, stroking, and talking softly help. The child just needs to know that he or she is loved and not fighting alone—reassurance over and over again is crucial to the child's peace of mind.
>
> He or she must also feel able to call on parents for help at any time during the night. The child needs some privacy—it's an embarrassing disease and he or she must be alone to cry or scratch or talk out loud—but must not feel *too* alone with his or her problem.
>
> In addition to verbal reassurances, the child needs a lot of physical contact. Touching cannot be overdone. Massage is perhaps the best way to communicate a physical acceptance of the child's body while soothing at the same time. Take care to touch the parts of the body that have been most affected by the eczema, even if your touch must be extremely gentle to avoid irritation.

Notes

Introduction

1. Grossbart (1982).

1. How This Book Can Help

1. See Edelson and Fink (1985) for a recent review.
2. Bartrop et al. (1977).
3. Reported in Goleman (1982).
4. See Locke and Colligan (1986) for a masterful review of the area.
5. Ikemi and Nakagawa (1962).
6. Not all of these attempts have been successful. Typically a doctor will have positive results with a previously successfully treated patient, then a more "scientific" approach, with college sophomores or other, much less interested and motivated subjects, will be unsuccessful. Crasilneck and Hall (1975); Chapman, Goodell and Wolff (1959).
7. Heilig and Hoff (1928).
8. Kaneko and Takaishi (1963).
9. See "Warts" in the Disease Directory.
10. Brown and Bettley (1971).
11. Crasilneck and Hall (1975) is a good summary of medical applications.
12. Porter et al. (1979).
13. *The Helper* (1981).
14. Nadelson (1978) and Griesemer and Nadelson (1979).
15. Van Keep (1976).

2. Listening to Your Skin

1. Spitz (1951).
2. All names are pseudonyms and where necessary some details have been altered to preserve confidentiality.
3. Frankel and Misch (1973). This case also provides a nice example of a team approach by two gifted therapists. Dr. Robert Misch did the psychotherapy and Dr. Fred Frankel the hypnotic work.
4. Scott (1960). This truly pioneering work is sadly long out of print. The publisher may provide photocopies.

3. "Why Me?" The Skin Has Its Reasons

1. Reich (1949) or various books by Alexander Lowen such as (1972).
2. The classic source is Freud (1953). Garfield (1976) is an exciting new approach that really works.
3. Freud (1953).
4. Ibid.
5. Deikman (1969).

5. Why Now?

1. Holmes and Rahe (1967).
2. See Toffler (1970) for a very readable review.
3. For more recent developments and controversies see Thoits.
4. See Griesemer and Nadelson (1979); and Griesemer (1978).
5. Davis and Bick (1946).

6. The Self-Sabotage Test

1. Obermeyer (1955).
2. Beare, Burrows, and Merrett (1978).
3. Shanon (1970) a, b, c.

7. Why There? Mapping Trouble Spots

1. Obermeyer, Witkauer and Edgell, quoted in Wittkower and Russell (1953).

8. What Your Symptom Does *for* You

1. A very good survey is Bresler (1979).

11. The Healing State: Your Untapped Resource

1. For more general background see Tart (1969) and Zinberg (1977).
2. See Benson 1975 and 1985.

3. For more reading on hypnosis and self-hypnosis, I suggest Frankel (1976), Bowers (1976), Fromm and Shor (1979), and Crasilneck and Hall (1975).

12. The Ideal Imaginary Environment: A Health Spa for Your Skin

1. For general background on imagery try Sheehan (1972) or Sheikh (1983).
2. Ikemi and Nakagawa (1962).
3. See Bresler (1979) for innovative uses of this technique.
4. While highly controversial, Simonton's (1978, 1984) work is a very useful resource.

13. Reinforcements: More Techniques to Help Now

1. Oyle (1975).
2. Bresler (1979).
3. Kroger (1963).

14. Thinking: Enemy or Ally

1. Shapiro (1965).
2. Cohant (1982).
3. Paulson and Petrus (1969) and Griesemer and Nadelson (1979).
4. Farber and Scott (1979).
5. For a sparkling application of the "cognitive therapy" techniques to depression see Burns (1980).

15. Biofeedback: The Electronic Doctor

1. Benson and Proctor (1984).
2. For more information on biofeedback see Aldine and Anchor.
3. Koldys and Meyer (1979).
4. Benoit and Harrell (1980).
5. Duller and Gentry (1980).
6. Brown (1981).

16. Psychotherapy: Help in Depth

1. Seitz (1953).
2. Brown and Bettley (1971).
3. Blank and Brody (1950).
4. Williams (1951).

17. Breaking the Itch-Scratch Cycle

1. See Appendix I for more of her story.
2. Fitzpatrick (1979).
3. Ibid.
4. Arndt (1984).

5. This is true of pain and though I have not seen enough patients with "medical" itching to conclude this directly, I think it a probable and useful idea.

6. See Brown and Kalucy (1975), and Tantam, Kalucy, and Brown (1982).

18. Holding On/Letting Go: Your Symptom's Last Stand

1. Greenson (1967).

19. Ghosts: Have They Handcuffed Your Doctors?

1. Freud (1912).
2. Again I have drawn on Greenson's (1967) classic work.

Disease Directory

1. For the basic description and conventional treatment of each disease I have used Fitzgerald (1979) and Arndt (1984).

For an older but very comprehensive and thoughtful summary of the psychological side of *any* skin problem, try to find a copy of Obermeyer (1955).

Whitlock (1976) is a more recent, quite comprehensive review. To my view he is unproductively cynical and hypercritical of psychological treatment. Use this book for information but don't be discouraged by it.

Wittkower and Russell (1953) is another useful general reference despite some unimpressive research techniques.

2. Fulton and Black (1983) is a very useful, readable, popular book.

Hirsch (1978) and Schacter et al. (1971) may be helpful to parents of adolescents.

Ellerbroek (1973) presents an intellectually challenging point of view—a unique contribution.

3. Ikemi & Nakagawa (1962).

4. Bray (1983).

5. Frazier (1977) a popular book.

6. Secter and Bathelemi (1964).

7. Jabush (1969).

8. Epstein et al. (1970).

9. See Wakeman and Kaplan (1978), and Crasilneck and Hall (1975).

10. See Locke (1986), LeShan (1959), Blumberg (1954), Krasnoff (1959), and Cooper (1985).

11. Simonton (1978).

12. LeShan (1959).

13. Rogentine et al. (1979).

14. Simonton (1978 and 1984).

15. Janicki (1971).
16. Wink (1966).
17. Spitz (1951).
18. Obermeyer (1955).
19. Wittkower and Russell (1953).
20. Griesemer and Nadelson (1979).
21. Twerski and Narr (1974), Brown and Bettley (1971), Miller and Coger (1979), and Cataldo (1980).
22. Hansen et al. (1981).
23. Ikemi and Nakagawa (1962).
24. Obermeyer (1955).
25. Ibid.
26. Kligman (1961).
27. Wittkower and Russell (1953).
28. Obermeyer (1955).
29. Melman and Griesemer (1968). For more adult information see Cohen and Lichtenberg (1967).
30. Oguchi and Miura (1977).
31. Sticher, Abramovits, and Newcomer (1980).
32. Oguchi and Miura (1977).
33. Galski (1981).
34. Langston (1983). This book is both the best general source and covers the widest variety of types and locations of herpes.
35. Heilig and Hoff (1929).
36. *The Helper* (1981).
37. Arone Di Bertolino (1981).
38. Gillespie (1982), Freudberg (1982), and Wickett (1982).
39. Langston (1983).
40. See Scott (1960) for this case and Obermeyer (1955) for other background. See also Langston (1983), a very well-done popular book.
41. Pistiner, Pitlik, Rosenfeld (1979), a brief report; Saul and Bernstein (1941) is a much richer source.
42. Kaneko and Takaishi (1963).
43. Werth (1978).
44. Graham and Wolf (1950).
45. Wittkower (1953).
46. Kaneko and Takaishi (1963).
47. Lerer (1977).
48. Kidd (1966) and Mason (1952).
49. Schneck (1954).
50. Obermeyer (1955).
51. Pollens (1986) is a very important and useful paper.
52. Arone Di Bertolino (1981).

53. Wilsch-Lieselotte and Hornstein (1976).
54. Thurn (1976).
55. Wilsch-Lieselotte and Hornstein (1976).
56. Shafi and Shafi (1979).
57. Seville (1978).
58. Stanker (1981).
59. Frankel and Misch (1973), Kline (1954), and Kohli (1967).
60. Coles (1967).
61. See Updike (1985) for an incise account of lifelong wrestling with psoriasis.
62. Wittkower and Russell (1953).
63. Scott (1960).
64. Wittkower and Russell (1953).
65. Griesemer and Nadelson (1979), Obermeyer (1955), Whitlak (1976), and Krupp (1977).
66. Obermeyer (1955), and Whitlock (1976).
67. Porter et al. (1979).
68. Gajwani and Sehgal (1974).
69. Rulinson (1942).
70. Ullman (1959), and Ullman and Dudek (1960) provide a good general review.
71. Surman et al. (1973) and Sinclair-Gieben (1959).
72. Owen Robbins, personal communication.
73. Ewing (1974), a very important paper. These warts are far more common than I had first realized and also predisposed to some cancers.

Appendix III: If Your Child Has the Problem

1. Fraiberg (1959) is a masterful portrayal of a child's reality.
2. Gardner and Oleness (1981) is an excellent overview of the potential of hypnosis with children.

Bibliography

Altered States of Consciousness, ed. Charles T. Tart. New York: Double-day, 1969.

Alternate States of Consciousness, ed. Norman E. Zinberg. New York: MacMillan, 1977.

American Journal of Clinical Biofeedback, ed. K. Auchor. New York: Human Sciences Press, periodical.

Arndt, K. A. *Manual of Dermatologic Therapeutics*, 3rd ed. Boston: Little Brown, 1983.

Arone Di Bertolino, R. "Terapia psicosomatica dell'herpes simplex recidivante," *Minerva Medica*, 72 (1981), 1207–1212.

————. "Hypnotherapy in a 22-month-old girl with molluscum contagiosum," *Minerva Medica*, 79 (1981), 1213–1215.

Bahnson, C. B., and M. B. Bahnson. "Role of the ego defenses: denial and repression in the etiology of malignant neoplasm," *Annals of the New York Academy of Science*, 123 (1966): 827–845.

Bartrop, R. W., et al. "Depressed Lymphocyte Function After Bereavement," *The Lancet*, 1 (1977), 834–836.

Beare, J. M., et al. "The effects of mental and physical stress on the incidence of skin disorders," *British Journal of Dermatology*, 98 (1978): 553–558.

Benoit, J., and E. H. Harrell. "Biofeedback and Control of Skin Cell Proliferation in Psoriasis," *Psychological Reports* (46), 1980: 831–839.

Benson, H. *The Relaxation Response*. New York: Morrow, 1975.

————, and W. Proctor. *Beyond the Relaxation Response: How to Harness the Healing Power of Your Personal Beliefs*. New York: Time, 1984.

Biofeedback and Self-Control (Annual), Chicago: Aldine.

Blank, H., and M. W. Brody. "Recurrent Herpes Simplex," *Psychosomatic Medicine*, 12 (1950), 254–260.

Blumberg, E. M., et al. "A possible relationship between psychological factors and human cancer," *Psychosomatic Medicine*, 16 (1954), 277–286.

Bowers, K. *Hypnosis for the Seriously Curious*, Montery, Calif.: Brooks-Cole, 1976.

Bray, S. Personal Communication (1983).

Bresler, D. E. *Free Yourself from Pain*. New York: Simon & Schuster, 1979.

Brown, B. W. "Treatment of Acne Vulgaris by Biofeedback-Assisted Cue-Controlled Relaxation and Guided Imagery," *Dissertation Abstracts International*, 42 (1981), 1163–B.

Brown, D. G., and F. R. Bettley. "Psychiatric Treatment of Eczema: A Controlled Trial," *British Medical Journal*, June 26, 1971, 729–734.

———, and R. S. Kalucy. "Correlation of Neurophysiological and Personality Data in Sleep Scratching," *Proceedings of the Royal Society of Medicine*, 68 (1975), 20–22.

Burns, D. D. *Feeling Good: The New Mood Therapy*. New York: Morrow, 1980.

Cataldo, M. F., et al. "Behavior Therapy Techniques in the Treatment of Exfoliative Dermatitis," *Archives of Dermatology*, 116 (1980), 919–922.

Chapman, L. F., et al. "Changes in Tissue Vulnerability During Hypnotic Suggestion," *Journal of Psychosomatic Research*, 4 (1959), 99–105.

Cohen, I., and J. D. Lichtenberg. "Alopecia Areata," *Archives of General Psychiatry*, 17 (1967), 608–614.

Coles, R. B. "Group Treatment in the Skin Department," *Transactions of the St. John's Hospital Dermatologic Society*, 53-1 (1967) 82–85.

Conant, Marcus A. Reported in "Instances of Delusional Genital Herpes Reported," *Clinical Psychiatry News*, 10–5, 1982, 29.

Crasilneck, H. B., and J. A. Hall. *Clinical Hypnosis Principles and Applications*. New York: Grune & Stratton, 1975.

Davis, D. B., and J. W. Bick. "Skin Reactions Observed Under War Time Stress," *Journal of Nervous and Mental Diseases*, 103 (1946), 503–508.

Deikman, A. J. "Deautomatization and the Mystical Experience," *Altered States of Consciousness*, ed. Charles T. Tart. New York: Doubleday, 1969.

Duller P., and W. D. Gentry. "Use of Biofeedback in Treating Chronic Hyperhidrosis: A Preliminary Report," *British Journal of Dermatology*, 103 (1980), 143–146.

Edelson, R. L., and J. M. Fink. "The Immunologic Function of Skin," *Scientific American*, 252-6 (1985), 44–53.

Epstein, E. S., et al. "Psychiatric Aspects of Behçet's Syndrome," *Journal of Psychosomatic Research*, 14 (1970), 161–172.

Farber E. M., and E. J. Van Scott. "Psoriasis," in *Dermatology in General Medicine*, eds. Fitzpatrick et al. New York: McGraw-Hill, 1979, 233–247.

Fitzpatrick, T. B. "Fundamentals of Dermatologic Diagnosis," *Dermatology in General Medicine*. New York: McGraw-Hill, 1979.

Flugel, J. *The Psychology of Clothes*, New York: AMS, 1930.

Fraiberg, S. *The Magic Years*, New York: Scribner's, 1959.

Frankel, Fred H. *Hypnosis: Trance as a Coping Mechanism*. New York: Plenum, 1976.

———, and R. C. Misch. "Hypnosis in a Case of Long-Standing Psoriasis in a Person with Character Problems," *The International Journal of Clinical and Experimental Hypnosis*, 21-3 (1973): 121–130.

Frazier, C. A. *Psychosomatic Aspects of Allergy*. New York: Van Nostrand, Reinhold, 1977.

Freud, S. "The Dynamics of Transference," in *The Standard Edition of the Complete Psychological Works of Sigmund Freud*. London: Hogarth, 1953, 97–108.

———. "The Interpretation of Dreams," in *The Standard Edition of the Complete Psychological Works of Sigmund Freud*, Vols. 4–5, ed. and trans. J. Strachey. London: Hogarth, 1953.

———. "The Psychopathology of Everyday Life," in *The Standard Edition of the Psychological Works of Sigmund Freud*, ed. and trans. J. Strachey. London: Hogarth, 1953.

Freudberg, F. *Herpes: A Complete Guide to Relief and Reassurance*. Philadelphia: Running Press, 1982.

Fulton, J. E., and E. Black. *Dr. Fulton's Step-by-Step Program for Clearing Acne*. New York: Harper & Row, 1983.

The Function and Nature of Imagery, ed. P. W. Sheehan. New York: Academic Press, 1972.

Gajwani, A. K., and V. N. Sehgal. "Hypnosis: A New Therapeutic Approach in Vitiligo," *Cutis*, 14 (1974): 572–573.

Galski, T. J. "The Adjunctive Use of Hypnosis in the Treatment of Trichotillomania: A Case Report," *American Journal of Clinical Hypnosis*, 23-3 (1981): 198–201.

Gardner, G. G., and K. Olness. *Hypnosis and Hypnotherapy with Children*, New York: Grune, 1981.

Garfield, P. *Creative Dreaming*. New York: Ballantine, 1976.

Gillespie, O. *Herpes: What to Do When You Have It*. New York: Grosset and Dunlap, 1982.

Bibliography

Goleman, D. "The Chicken Soup Effect," *Psychology Today*, December 1982: 81–82.

Graham, D. T., and S. Wolf. "Pathogenesis of Urticaria," *Journal of the American Medical Association*, 143 (1950), 1396–1402.

Greenson, R. R. *The Technique and Practice of Psychoanalysis*. New York: International Universities Press, 1967.

Griesemer, R. D. "Emotionally Triggered Disease in a Dermatological Practice," *Psychiatric Annals*, 8:8 (1978): 49–56.

————, and T. Nadelson. "Emotional Aspects of Cutaneous Disease," in *Dermatology in General Medicine*, T. B. Fitzpatrick et al. New York: McGraw-Hill, 1979, 1353–1363.

Grossbart, T. A. "Bringing Peace to Embattled Skin," *Psychology Today*, 16-2 (1982), 54–60.

Hansen, O. et al. "My Fingers Itch but My Hands Are Bound: An Exploratory Psychosomatic Study of Patients with Dyshidrosis of the Hands," *Zeitschrift Fur Psychosomatische Medizin und Psychoanalyse*, 27-3 (1981), 275–290.

Heilig, R., and H. Hoff. *"Uberpsychogene Entstehung des Herpes Labialis,"* *Medizinische Klinik*, 24: 1472 (1928).

"HELP Membership HSV Survey Research Project Results," *The Helper*, 3:2 (1981), 1–5.

Hirsch, J. G. "Understanding the Adolescent Patient," *Major Problems in Clinical Pediatrics*, 19 (1978), 28–38.

Holmes, T. H., and R. H. Rahe. "The Social Readjustment Rating Scale," *Journal of Psychosomatic Research*, 11 (1967), 213–218.

Hypnosis: Developments in Research and New Perspectives. eds. E. Fromm and R. E. Shor.

Ikemi, Y., and S. Nakagawa. "A Psychosomatic Study of Contagious Dermatitis," *Kyushu Journal of Medical Science*, 13 (1962), 335–350.

Imagery: Current Theory, Research, and Application, ed. A. A. Sheikh. New York: Wiley & Sons, 1983.

Jabush, M. "A Case of Chronic Recurring Multiple Boils Treated with Hypnotherapy," *Psychiatric Quarterly*, 43-3 (1969), 448–455.

Janicki, M. P. "Recurrent Herpes Labialis and Recurrent Apthous Ulcerations: Psychological Components," *Psychotherapy and Psychosomatics*, 19 (1971), 288–294.

Kaneko, Z., and N. Takaishi. "Psychosomatic Studies on Chronic Urticaria," *Folia Psychiatrica et Neurologica Japonica*, 17-1 (1963), 16–24.

Kidd, C. B. "Congenital Ichthyosiform Erythroderma Treated by Hypnosis," *British Journal of Dermatology*, 78 (1966), 101.

Kligman, A. M. "Pathologic Dynamics of Human Hair Loss," *Archives of Dermatology*, 83 (1961), 175.

Kline, M. V. "Psoriasis and Hypnotherapy: A Case Report," *Journal of Clinical and Experimental Hypnosis*, 2 (1954), 318–323.

Kohli, D. R. "Psoriasis: A Physiopathologic Adaptive Reaction," *Northwest Medicine*, January 1967, 33–39.

Koldys, K. W., and R. P. Meyer. "Biofeedback Training in the Therapy of Dyshidrosis," *Cutis*, 24 (1979), 219–221.

Krasnoff, A. "Psychological Variables and Human Cancer: A Cross-Validation Study," *Psychosomatic Medicine*, 21 (1959), 291–295.

Kroger, W. S. *Clinical and Experimental Hypnosis*. Philadelphia: J. B. Lippincott, 1963.

Krupp, N. E. "Self-Caused Skin Ulcers," *Psychosomatics*, 18 (1977), 15–19.

Langston, D. P. *Living with Herpes*. New York: Dolphin, 1983.

Lerer, B. "Hyperhidrosis: A Review of Its Psychological Aspects," *Psychosomatics*, 18-5 (1977), 28–31.

LeShan, L. "Psychological States as Factors in the Development of Malignant Disease: A Critical Review," *Journal of the National Cancer Institute*, 22 (1959), 1–18.

Locke, S., and D. Colligan. *The Healer Within: The New Medicine of Mind and Body*. New York: Dutton, 1986.

Lowen, A. *The Betrayal of the Body*. New York: Collier, 1972.

Mason, A. A. "Case of Congenital Ichthyosiform Erythrodermia of Brocq Treated by Hypnosis," *British Medical Journal*, 2 (1952), 422.

Mehlman, R. D., and R. D. Griesemer. "Alopecia Areata in the Very Young," *American Journal of Psychiatry*, 125 (1968), 57–65.

Miller, R. M., and R. W. Coger. "Skin conductance conditioning with dyshidrotic eczema patients," *British Journal of Dermatology*, 101 (1979): 435–440.

Nadelson, T. "A Person's Boundaries: A Meaning of Skin Disease," *Cutis*, 21 (1978), 90–94.

Obermayer, M. E. *Psychocutaneous Medicine*. Springfield, Ill.: Charles C. Thomas, 1955.

Oguchi, T., and S. Miura. "Trichotillomania: Its Psychopathological Aspect," *Comprehensive Psychiatry*, 18 (1977), 177–182.

Oyle, I. *The Healing Mind*. Berkeley, Calif.: Celestial Arts, 1975.

Paulson, M. J., and E. P. Petrus. "Delusions of Parasitosis: A Psychological Study," *Psychosomatics*, 10 (1969), 111–120.

Pistner, M., et al. "Psychogenic Urticaria," *The Lancet*, 22/29 (1979), 1383.

Pollens, M. S. "Ericksonian Hypnosis and Psychoanalytic Psychotherapy: The Anatomy of an Effective Partnership in the Clinical Management of Auto-Immune Disease," *Journal of Contemporary Psychotherapy*, 15-2 (1986).

Porter, J., et al. "Psychological Reaction to Chronic Skin Disorders: A Study of Patients with Vitiligo," *General Hospital Psychiatry* (1979), 73–77.

Psychosocial Stress and Cancer, ed. C. L. Cooper. New York: Wiley, 1985.

Reich, Wilhelm. *Character Analysis*. New York: Farrar, Straus and Giroux, 1949.

Rogentine, G. N., et al. "Psychosocial Factors in the Prognosis of Malignant Melanoma: A Prospective Study," *Psychosomatic Medicine*, 41 (1979), 647–655.

Rulinson, R. H. "Warts: A Statistical Study of 921 Cases," *Archives of Dermatology and Syphilology*, 46 (1942), 66–81.

Saul, L. J., and C. Bernstein. "The Emotional Settings of Some Attacks of Urticaria," *Psychosomatic Medicine* 3 (1941), 349–369.

Schachter, R. J., et al. "Acne Vulgaris and Psychological Impact on High School Students," *New York State Journal of Medicine* (1971), 2886–2890.

Schneck, J. M. "Ichthyosis Treated with Hypnosis," *Diseases of the Nervous System*, 15 (1954), 211.

Scott, Michael J. *Hypnosis in Skin and Allergic Diseases*. Springfield, Ill.: Charles C. Thomas, 1960.

Secter, I. I., and C. G. Barthelemy. "Angular Cheilosis and Psoriasis as Psychosomatic Manifestations," *American Journal of Clinical Hypnosis*, 7 (1964), 79–81.

Seitz, P. F. D. "Dynamically Oriented Brief Psychotherapy: Psychocutaneous Excoriation Syndromes," *Psychosomatic Medicine*, 15 (1953), 200–242.

Seville, R. H. "Psoriasis and Stress," *British Journal of Dermatology*, 98 (1978), 151–153.

Shafi, M., and S. L. Shafi. "Exploratory Psychotherapy in the Treatment of Psoriasis, Twelve Hundred Years Ago," *Archives of General Psychiatry*, 36 (1979), 1242–1245.

Shanon, J. "Delayed Psychosomatic Skin Disorders in Survivors of Concentration Camps," *British Journal of Dermatology*, 83 (1970), 536–542.

———. "Psychosomatic Skin Disorders in Survivors of Nazi Concentration Camps," *Psychosomatics*, 11-2 (1970), 95–98.

———. "The Subconscious Motivation for the Appearance of Psychosomatic Skin Disorders in Concentration Camp Survivors and Their Rehabilitation," *Psychosomatics*, 11-3 (1970), 178–182.

Shapiro, D. *Neurotic Styles*. New York: Basic, 1965.

Simonton, O. C., et al. *Getting Well Again*. Los Angeles: J. P. Tarcher, Inc., 1978.

Simonton, S., and R. Shook. *Healing Family*. New York: Bantam, 1984.

Sinclair-Gieben, A. H. C., and D. Chalmers. "Evaluation of Treatment of Warts by Hypnosis," *The Lancet*, 10/3 (1959), 480–482.

Spitz, R. A. "The Psychogenic Diseases of Infancy," *Psychoanalytic Study of Child*, 6 (1951), 255–275.

Stanker, L. "The Effect of Psoriasis on the Sufferer," *Clinical and Experimental Dermatology*, 5/6-3 (1981), 303–306.

Sticher, M., et al. "Trichotillomania in Adults," *Cutis*, 26 (1980), 90–101.

Surman, O. S., et al. "Hypnosis in the Treatment of Warts," *Archives of General Psychiatry*, 28 (1973), 439–441.

Tantum, D., et al. "Sleep, Scratching and Dreams in Eczema: A New Approach to Alexithymia," *Psychotherapy and Psychosomatics*, 37 (1982), 26–35.

Tasini, M. F., and T. P. Hackett. "Hypnosis in the Treatment of Warts in Immunodeficient Children," *American Journal of Clinical Hypnosis*, 19-3 (1977), 152–154.

Thoits, P. A. "Social Support Processes and Psychological Well-being: Theoretical Possibilities," in *Social Support: Theory, Research and Application*, eds. I. G. Sarason and B. R. Sarason. The Hague, the Netherlands: Martinus Nijhof.

Thurn, A. "Psychogenic Aspects of Perioral Dermatitis," *Zeitschrift fur Psychosomatische Medizin und Psychoanalyse*, 22-1 (1976), 99–109.

Toffler, A. *Future Shock*. New York: Random House, 1970.

Twerski, A. J., and R. Narr. "Hypnotherapy in a Case of Refractory Dermatitis," *American Journal of Clinical Hypnosis*, 16-3 (1974), 202–205.

Ullman, M. "On the Psyche and Warts," *Psychosomatic Medicine*, 21-6 (1959), 473–488.

———, and S. Dudek. "On the Psyche and Warts," *Psychosomatic Medicine*, 22-1 (1960), 67–76.

Updike, J. "Personal History: At War with My Skin," *The New Yorker*, September 2, 1985.

Van Keep, P. A. "Isolation: The influence of skin disease on social relationships," *International Journal of Dermatology*, 15 (1976): 446–449.

Wakeman, R. J., and J. Z. Kaplan. "An Experimental Study of Hypnosis in Painful Burns," *American Journal of Clinical Hypnosis*, 21 (1978), 3–12.

Werth, G. R. "The Hives Dilemma," *American Family Physician*, 17 (1978), 139–143.

Whitlock, F. A. *Psychophysiological Aspects of Skin Disease*. London: Saunders, 1976.

Wickett, W. H. *Herpes: Cause and Control*. New York: Pinnacle, 1982.

Williams, D. H. "Management of Atopic Dermatitis in Children: Control of the Maternal Rejection Factor," *Archives of Dermatology*, 63 (1951), 545–560.

Wilsch, L., and O. P. Hornstein. "Statistical Studies and Results of

Treatment of Patients with Perioral Dermatitis," *Zeitschrift fur Psychosomatische Medizin und Psychoanalyse*, 22 (1976), 115–125.

Wink, C. A. S. "A Case of Darier's Disease Treated by Hypnotic Age Regression," *American Journal of Hypnosis*, 9-2 (1966), 146–150.

Wittkower, E. "Studies of the Personality of Patients Suffering from Urticaria," *Psychosomatic Medicine*, 15 (1953), 177.

———, and B. Russell. *Emotional Factors in Skin Disease*. New York: Hoeber, 1953.

Index

ABOUT THE AUTHORS

Dr. Ted Grossbart is a clinical psychologist in private practice affiliated with Beth Israel Hospital in Boston, and is a member of the faculty of Harvard Medical School. The techniques of self-help he teaches in *Skin Deep* were perfected over his many years' experience in private practice, treating patients suffering the mental and physical torments of skin disease. He is a Phi Beta Kappa graduate of the University of Michigan and received his M.A. and Ph.D. in clinical psychology from Boston University.

Dr. Grossbart lives with his wife, Rosely Traube, also a clinical psychologist, and their two sons, Zachary and Matthew, in Marblehead, Massachusetts.

Carl Sherman graduated from Harvard College and received his Ph.D. from Harvard University. He has been the executive editor of *Executive Fitness Newsletter* and a senior editor of *Prevention* magazine. One of the best science writers in the field, Carl Sherman's articles have appeared in *Glamour*, *McCall's*, *Science Digest*, and *Vital*.